THE HEALTHCARE PROFESSIONAL WORKFORCE

The Healthcare Professional Workforce

UNDERSTANDING HUMAN CAPITAL IN A CHANGING INDUSTRY

Edited by
Timothy J. Hoff

PROFESSOR OF MANAGEMENT, HEALTHCARE SYSTEMS, AND HEALTH POLICY
PATRICK AND HELEN WALSH RESEARCH PROFESSOR
D'AMORE-MCKIM SCHOOL OF BUSINESS
SCHOOL OF PUBLIC POLICY AND URBAN AFFAIRS
NORTHEASTERN UNIVERSITY
VISITING ASSOCIATE FELLOW, OXFORD UNIVERSITY

Kathleen M. Sutcliffe

BLOOMBERG DISTINGUISHED PROFESSOR OF BUSINESS AND MEDICINE
CAREY BUSINESS SCHOOL
SCHOOL OF MEDICINE
JOHNS HOPKINS UNIVERSITY

Gary J. Young

DIRECTOR, NORTHEASTERN UNIVERSITY CENTER FOR HEALTH POLICY
  AND HEALTHCARE RESEARCH
PROFESSOR OF STRATEGIC MANAGEMENT AND HEALTHCARE SYSTEMS
D'AMORE-MCKIM SCHOOL OF BUSINESS AND BOUVÉ COLLEGE
  OF HEALTH SCIENCES
NORTHEASTERN UNIVERSITY

OXFORD
UNIVERSITY PRESS

OXFORD
UNIVERSITY PRESS

Oxford University Press is a department of the University of Oxford. It furthers
the University's objective of excellence in research, scholarship, and education
by publishing worldwide. Oxford is a registered trade mark of Oxford University
Press in the UK and certain other countries.

Published in the United States of America by Oxford University Press
198 Madison Avenue, New York, NY 10016, United States of America.

© Oxford University Press 2017

Library of Congress Cataloging-in-Publication Data
Names: Hoff, Timothy J., 1965– , editor. | Sutcliffe, Kathleen M., 1950– , editor. | Young, Gary J., editor.
Title: The healthcare professional workforce : Understanding human capital in a changing industry /
[edited by] Timothy J. Hoff, Kathleen M. Sutcliffe, Gary J. Young.
Description: Oxford ; New York : Oxford University Press, [2016] | Description based on print version
record and CIP data provided by publisher; resource not viewed.
Identifiers: LCCN 2016008601 (print) | LCCN 2016007431 (ebook) | ISBN 9780190215668 |
ISBN 9780190215675 | ISBN 9780190215651 (pbk. : alk. paper)
Subjects: | MESH: Health Occupations—trends | Allied Health Personnel—trends | Health Care
Reform—organization & administration | United States
Classification: LCC R697.A4 (print) | LCC R697.A4 (ebook) | NLM W 21 | DDC 610.73/7069—dc23
LC record available at http://lccn.loc.gov/2016008601

9 8 7 6 5 4 3 2 1
Printed by Webcom, Inc., Canada

Contents

Preface

THE IDEA FOR this book came from our own view that much is happening to the various health professions in the early 21st century. This is particularly true in the United States. Nationwide health reform, combined with continued problems of inflation, quality, and access in the healthcare industry, has created an everyday work environment for physicians, nurses, and other medical professionals that upends traditional notions about what it means to be a certain type of health professional, the types of work and autonomy afforded various expert workers, and the substance of professional relationships with fellow workers and corporate organizations that now control much of American healthcare. In these regards, and in other ways, it is a transformative time for health professions in the United States. This book's motivation derives from a sense that it is an ideal time for examining some of the important trends, issues, and opportunities that affect health professionals. It is equally important to analyze how these workers and contexts will evolve into the future.

In all the upheaval around the healthcare system, the professionals who work in it often get the least attention. This observation points to something ironic in healthcare research, management, and policymaking—that those individuals who perform the bulk of the work of healthcare seem to have less voice and command less attention than is warranted. Thus, new payment systems are designed and implemented with little regard for what physicians think may work to improve how they deliver care; scopes of work for nurses and pharmacists are expanded without much consideration of what these new opportunities mean for their relationships with physicians, patients, and their employers; and entire swaths of healthcare work are redesigned for "efficiency" with less understanding of whether the professionals in those workflows will respond in desirable ways. This book seeks in small part to correct this oversight. By placing physicians, nurses, pharmacists, physician assistants, and others center stage, we hope to encourage healthcare academics, policymakers, practitioners, educators, and students to pay more attention to these groups in the future.

That said, there are important realities all health professionals face that will not go away any time soon. These realities require both a rethinking and reexamination of important issues such as professional training, professional belief systems, professional–organizational alignment, professional diversity, leading professionals, professional scopes of practice, talent management of professionals, and interprofessional collaboration. These are the kinds of issues addressed in this book. We are fortunate to have contributing authors who are leading experts on the health professions. They have done a terrific job in unpacking some of these issues for us. Our intention is to address issues not only critical for the present and near future, but also ones that affect multiple professional groups in healthcare. Although the book includes distinct chapters that focus on the medical profession and certain types of other health professionals, the remainder of the book discusses different issues with a variety of health professions in mind.

If readers learn something new, or reflect differently on their existing knowledge by reading this volume, then we believe that our mission has been accomplished. As an incomplete dive into the world of US health professional change, the work is not meant as the full and final word on US health professions change. Rather, it is a reference for moving certain existing discussions along, for starting others, in the meantime pushing the health professional agenda further into the mainstream of healthcare education, policy, management, and research. We believe that there is no more important time for thinking about health professions than now. This means considering everything from how we conceptualize and build theory around these expert workers, to how we train and study them, and to how to organize and manage their work. The book is written in an accessible way to allow different audiences a chance to get something out of it useful for themselves. Toward that end, we have also tried to limit jargon, make abstract ideas more practically focused, and stay on point with specific themes that thread throughout the book. Ultimately, readers can judge if we have achieved these goals.

Timothy J. Hoff
Kathleen M. Sutcliffe
Gary J. Young
February, 2016

Acknowledgments

Every book is a labor of love, and edited books present additional challenges of achieving coordination among different and often very busy authors, cajoling these authors to meet tight timelines, and then bringing the different voices together to make a coherent whole. That said such books are not possible without the dedication of individuals who give of their time and intellectual capital so that a given scholarly area can be further illuminated for a reading audience. We would like to thank all of the authors who contributed to this volume. They are leaders in their respective fields who thought it worthwhile to contribute around the topic of the health professions workforce. We are all fortunate that they made this decision.

Our academic institutions (Northeastern University, Johns Hopkins University) also deserve sincere thanks. They both are outstanding settings in which to engage in high-level scholarship. The three of us benefit from being given the time and support to develop and bring to fruition projects such as this one. Both institutions have a rich history of training a variety of health care professionals, so it is fitting that this volume has emanated from these two places. As health professions continue to transform, these universities and the others to which our co-authors belong, as well as the professional associations and delivery systems led by several of our commentators, will no doubt remain on the cutting edge of innovation. That is encouraging to know.

Our debts to one another as co-editors also must be acknowledged. A lot of time and effort was put into this work. There were times during the process when the kinds of decisions we had to make, the editorial imperatives, and our own writing of chapters made compilation of the volume a complex endeavor. However, we are optimistic that the book will make a meaningful contribution to the field, and be an interesting read to several different audiences, and that feeling makes the effort we gave worthwhile. Our colleagues at Oxford University Press, specifically our editor Chad Zimmerman and his assistant Chloe Layman, have been tremendous resources for us, consistently helpful, and definitely made it much easier to pull this all together.

Finally, there are thanks which are more personal. For one co-editor (T.H.), the constant love and support of his wife Sharon and eight-year old son Kieran make everything in life easier and more worthwhile. Another co-editor (K.S.) knows that none of this would be possible without the loving patience and support of her family, especially Tim Wintermute. The remaining co-editor (G.Y.) is deeply thankful for the love and support of his family, wife Andrea, and children Samantha and Spencer.

We hope readers enjoy the book, and gain something useful from it. In preparing it, we believed (and still do) that there is nothing quite like it right now in the scholarly marketplace. The focus on multiple health professions, blend of different experts writing about these various professions, and the incorporation of important topics including training, talent management, organizational integration, leadership, and diversity make for a great primer on health professions change. Undoubtedly, the volume raises more questions than it answers. But then that is our intent—to have a work like this stimulate further dialogue around issues to which our response as a society will shape the kind of health care system we have for years to come.

Timothy J. Hoff
Kathleen M. Sutcliffe
Gary J. Young
July 2016

Contributors

Jeffrey A. Alexander, PhD
Richard Carl Jelinek Professor of
  Health Management and Policy
Professor, Organizational Behavior
  and Human Resources
School of Business
University of Michigan

Lawton Robert Burns, PhD, MBA
James Joo-Jin Kim Professor
Director, Wharton Center for Health
  Management and Economics
The Wharton School
University of Pennsylvania

James F. Cawley, PA-C, MPH
Professor, Department of
  Community Health
Professor, Department of Physician
  Assistant Studies
Milken Institute School of Public Health
The George Washington University

**Patricia M. Davidson, PhD, MEd,
RN, FAAN**
Professor and Dean, School of Nursing
Johns Hopkins University

Alan Dow, MD, MSHA
Assistant Vice President,
  Interprofessional Education
  and Collaborative Care
Professor, Internal Medicine
Virginia Commonwealth University

Lynne Eickholt, MBA
Chief Strategy Officer, Partners
  HealthCare System

Darrell G. Kirch, MD
President and Chief Executive Officer,
  Association of American Medical
  Colleges

Ralph W. Muller, MA
Chief Executive Officer, University
of Pennsylvania Health System

Mirko Noordegraaf, PhD
Head, Utrecht University School
of Governance
Professor, Utrecht University School
of Governance

Henry Pohl, MD
Vice Dean for Academic
Administration
Julio A. Sosa, MD, Chair of Medical
Education
Albany Medical College

Scott Reeves, PhD, MSc, PGCE
Professor in Interprofessional Research
at the Faculty of Health,
Social Care & Education
Kingston University & St George's,
University of London
Editor-in-Chief, Journal of
Interprofessional Care

Jon Schommer, PhD
Peters Chair in Pharmacy Practice
Innovation
Associate Department Head
and Professor, Department
of Pharmaceutical Care and
Health System
College of Pharmacy
University of Minnesota

Joanne Spetz, PhD
Professor, Institute of Health
Policy Studies
Professor, Department of Family
and Community Medicine
University of California, San Francisco

George Thibault, MD
President, Josiah Macy Jr. Foundation

1

INTRODUCTION TO THE BOOK AND THE FORCES

TRANSFORMING THE HEALTH PROFESSIONAL

WORKFORCE IN THE UNITED STATES

*Timothy J. Hoff, Kathleen M. Sutcliffe, and Gary J. Young**

Introduction

In this first chapter, we discuss the myriad of sweeping developments that are transforming the US health professional workforce. The health professional workforce itself is both large and diverse, comprising physicians, nurses, pharmacists, therapists (e.g., physical therapists, speech pathologists), dentists, podiatrists, physician assistants, and others. Based on data compiled by the federal government's National Center for Health Workforce Analysis, more than 5 million individuals currently work as health professionals in the United States (National Center for Health Workforce Analysis, 2013). This number is growing, and reflects an increasing diversity of jobs, employment settings, work arrangements, training, and personal expectations.

Both the makeup and expertise of various health professional groups are changing as a result of various healthcare reform initiatives, innovations in serving patients, changing patient attitudes toward healthcare services and efforts within various health professions to advance their specific claims to new or evolving forms of healthcare work. Although some of the developments that are transforming the health professions workforce have been in motion for some time, until quite recently the settings within which this workforce performed were relatively stable. A variety

*All authors contributed equally and are listed alphabetically.

of health professionals with circumscribed roles worked within well-defined patient care work domains so that little competition for patients existed among them. For example, within healthcare delivery organizations such as hospitals and ambulatory care practices, the decision-making authority of physicians for patient care was both well established and largely unchallenged, and other health professionals functioned largely in supporting roles. Health professionals were paid in ways that rewarded them for "good work" that was largely centered on patient volume rather than quality of care. Patients' engagement in their own healthcare was relatively limited, enabling health professionals to largely determine when, where, and what services should be delivered, often in a more paternalistic way. Health professionals of all types were trained independently of any recognition that their work should be collaborative and interdisciplinary. Workflows within service delivery organizations moved at a pace physicians determined.

Much has changed over the past two decades. For example, the country's expansive health reform law, the Patient Protection and Affordable Care Act, has been an important catalyst for change within the health professions, helping to accelerate trends begun years earlier as a result of the modern quality movement, managed care, and the growing corporatization of healthcare delivery. Underlying key developments affecting the health professions are noble goals—the country's long-standing struggle to contain healthcare costs, improve quality of care, and expand access to healthcare services. These struggles have provoked much soul-searching within the country in terms of what we can and should expect from our health professionals in terms of patient care and their own contributions to improving the system on these different fronts. It has also unleashed structural and cultural changes within health professional groups that require profound reexamination such as professional training and socialization, intraprofessional relationships, professional autonomy, and the alignment of health professionals with organizations.

The remainder of this chapter highlights some of the key developments driving professional change in healthcare. It is not intended as an exhaustive list but rather an overview of the most important contextual issues now occurring that have an impact on professionals.

Changes in How Healthcare is Organized, Managed, and Reimbursed

The increased standardization of care in the United States is a profound change that has been occurring for the past several decades. Care standardization has its origins in the evidence-based medicine movement of the 1970s and 1980s, found greater traction during the managed care era in the 1990s, and has been legitimized as rational response to the need to improve quality and lower healthcare costs in the United States (Timmermans, 2005). Numerous studies demonstrate substantial variation in treatment approaches among providers, particularly physicians, for patients with the same clinical condition (e.g., Birkmeyer, Sharp, Finlayson, Fisher, & Wennberg, 1998; Baicker, Buckles, & Chandra, 2006; Dubois, Batchlor, & Wade, 2002; Baker, Fisher, & Wennberg, 2008). It is now well established that providers' treatment choices vary geographically and in relation to other factors that are unrelated to medical evidence. Policymakers and health policy experts view these treatment variations as a major source of inefficiency and poor quality of care (Timmermans, 2005). Several initiatives in particular have been undertaken to reduce unwarranted variations in treatment approaches.

One key care standardization initiative has been the development and dissemination of clinical guidelines or protocols. Guidelines are explicit recommendations, generally grounded in available scientific evidence, for either selecting a treatment or managing a clinical condition (Cabana et al., 1999; Timmermans, 2005). As such, they constitute decision rules that are intended to reflect best practices for treating a clinical condition or performing a procedure. The use of standardized guidelines now dominates large segments of American healthcare, in particular around chronic disease management. Thousands of guidelines have been produced by government agencies, professional societies, and research organizations (Timmermans, 2005). Some guidelines address the clinical activities of physicians exclusively, but many others cover the clinical roles and responsibilities of various health professions relative to the management of patients for a specific diagnosis such as diabetes or procedures such as joint replacement. As health plans and other purchasers of healthcare services have adopted these guidelines for their own internal policies, the guidelines have become key benchmarks for assessing providers' quality of care and, increasingly, as justification for paying them.

Another initiative related to guideline development pertains to health information technologies, namely decision support systems, electronic medical records, and computerized physician order entry systems (CPOE). These technologies are often designed to promote providers' compliance with explicit treatment recommendations or decision rules when they use the technology to enter and access clinical information. For example, CPOEs will typically guide the prescriber regarding the selection and dosage of a medication following the entry of a specific set of clinical criteria (Grossman, Gerland, Reed, & Fahlman, 2007; Metzger, Welebob, Bates, Lipsitz, & Classen, 2010).

Process improvement activities, which include a family of approaches such as total quality management, continuous quality improvement, and reengineering constitute another care standardization initiative (e.g., Cima et al., 2011). Although these process improvement activities differ somewhat in their principles and methods, they generally focus on reducing performance variation for patient care activities through identifying and institutionalizing best practices. They also emphasize a systems perspective for improving patient care that highlights the role of processes rather than people as factors driving unwarranted variation in patient care practices (Sollecito & Johnson, 2012).

Guidelines and other efforts to standardize patient care have been greeted with mixed reactions by health professionals. While some have applauded the efforts, others have derisively referred to them as "cook book medicine" (Timmermans, 2005; Buchman et al., 2006). Advocates emphasize that these initiatives can improve providers' decision-making by distilling often vast amounts of clinical information into more manageable choice sets. Among detractors, some of the opposition reflects concerns that standardization weakens the clinical autonomy of health professionals and thus reduces their influence and prestige within the domain of patient care. But additional and legitimate concerns also exist that guidelines all too often rely on flimsy evidence and/or may fail to acknowledge important exceptions or contraindications to their recommendations (Buchman et al., 2006).

Professionals also lament that guidelines are not helpful in situations where the unique aspects of a patient's situation have an impact on health and, in fact may do more harm than good in encouraging the provider to ignore a detailed physical and history examination process. Moreover, studies examining the impact of health information technologies on patient outcomes have produced largely mixed results (e.g., Eslami, Abu-Hanna, & de Keizer et al., 2007; Buntin, Burke, Hoaglin, & Blumenthal, 2011). Providers have often found these technologies cumbersome to use and workarounds appear common (Grossman et al., 2007; Mitka, 2009). Furthermore, according to at least some research, organizations often implement process improvement initiatives in ways that suggest they are more interested in external legitimacy than identifying effective ways to deliver patient care (Westphal, Gulati, & Shortell, 1997; Young, Charns, & Shortell, 2001).

Nevertheless, efforts to standardize care will continue as unexplained treatment variations continue to persist (Weinstein, Bronner, Morgan, & Wennberg, 2004; Institute of Medicine, 2013). For health professionals, efforts to standardize care have helped usher in an era of external oversight and control over their activities that is displacing long-standing professional self-regulation (Marmor & Gordon, 2014). This presents a challenge to health professionals regarding how to maintain their influence over patient care. For many health professionals in the future, opportunities for autonomy may come in a "softer" form through leadership roles on the decision-making bodies that have responsibility for developing and implementing guidelines and other standardized forms of clinical decision-making (Levay & Waks, 2009).

Another key development for health professionals, particularly physicians, involves ongoing efforts to reform how they will be reimbursed for patient care. Historically, providers, both individuals and organizations, have been paid on a fee-for-service basis whereby payment was unrelated to service quality or efficiency. This is changing as public and private purchasers of healthcare services are moving to pay providers, particularly physicians and hospitals, in ways that link payment to predefined performance metrics for patient care. The mantra among purchasers is "pay for value, not volume." The new methods for payment, known generally as pay-for-performance (P4P) or value-based purchasing, build on previously discussed standardization initiatives because many of the performance metrics included in these payment arrangements typically comprise clinical guidelines and explicitly defined measures (Young, 2013; Friedberg et al., 2015).

These new payment methods vary in their specific designs. In particular, some P4P methods are integrated into existing fee-for-service arrangements whereby providers have financial incentives to achieve performance targets for either quality, efficiency, or both. By contrast, some purchasers are moving away from fee-for-service arrangements entirely in favor of capitated or global payment models. In these alternative payment models, providers receive a fixed budget for assuming responsibility for the care of either a defined population of patients (i.e., global budget) or an interrelated set of services that might correspond, for example, to a clinical procedure (i.e., bundled payments). As such, providers are incentivized to perform efficiently to remain within the given budget but typically have additional financial incentives under these payment arrangements for achieving quality-related performance targets (Friedberg et al., 2015).

P4P is growing in importance as a way of reimbursing professionals such as physicians. The Patient Protection and Affordable Care Act (PPACA), the country's sweeping healthcare reform law, authorized several such programs for Medicare, the federal insurance program for seniors. A P4P program for hospitals was rolled out in 2012. In 2015, a P4P program was rolled out for large physician practices. The law also authorized several demonstration or pilot programs for nursing homes and other types of provider organizations. Senior officials of the Centers for Medicare and Medicaid Services, the federal agency that administers Medicare, announced that by 2018, 90% of provider payments will be linked to performance metrics for quality and efficiency and 50% of payments will be made through alternative payment arrangements (Burwell, 2015). Most states now include P4P designs in their Medicaid programs. Also, hundreds of private-sector health plans throughout the country have established P4P programs for hospitals and physicians. According to one estimate, approximately 40% of commercial sector payments to physicians and hospitals are now linked to performance-based criteria for quality and efficiency (Delbanco, 2014).

Payment reform may have important implications for health professionals in terms of their work and professional identity. Like the previously noted initiatives to standardize healthcare, P4P is aimed at promoting providers' compliance with performance standards and effectively seeks to impose controls over their clinical decision-making. But unlike pure standardization approaches, P4P explicitly links compliance with payment as a motivational device. For many physicians, these new payment methods directly affect how they are paid for their work. For other health professionals such as nurses and pharmacists, who are more likely to be salaried employees of healthcare organizations that are reimbursed under these new payment methods, they are affected indirectly as the organizations that employ them consider how to best manage such professions to achieve organization-wide efficiency and quality goals. For some organizations, this may entail restructuring the traditional salary arrangements of health professionals to include more incentive-based pay linked to predefined efficiency and quality metrics that align with those of the organization's (Friedberg et al., 2015). It may also mean restructuring professional work and jobs in ways that upset the established order.

Various economic and psychological theories support the application of P4P to healthcare settings (Conrad & Perry 2009; Young, Beckman, & Baker, 2012). However, certain theoretical perspectives also raise warning signs that such payment programs will prove futile or even detrimental to the goal of efficient, high-quality care. For example, from the standpoint of self-determination theory (Ryan & Deci, 2000), financial incentives may cause health professionals to feel manipulated, leading them to find ways to game incentive systems strictly for their own benefit. Although the long-term effects of using financial incentives in healthcare are not yet clear, the numerous studies that have evaluated the short-term effects of P4P programs have generally found at best modest gains in providers' performance (Christianson, Leatherman, & Sutherland, 2008; Van Herck et al., 2010; Petersen et al., 2013; Benzer et al., 2014). Still, we are only beginning to gain the necessary experience to assess how incentive-based payments may affect the mindset and behavior of health professionals.

Another of the many changes that health professionals are experiencing involves the basic structures through which care is organized and delivered. For much of the twentieth century, healthcare was a cottage industry because most services were delivered through traditional service models that featured the independence of providers. The great majority of physicians worked in solo or small practices. Other health professionals such as nurses and therapists worked as employees of healthcare delivery organizations such as hospitals and nursing homes that operated as distinct and independent facilities.

During the past 25 years, the US healthcare industry has undergone consolidation as hospitals, physician organizations, and other types of providers have come together to form increasingly complex delivery systems through asset acquisitions and strategic alliances. Although providers involved in these consolidation efforts have almost always presented them to the public as a means to improve efficiency through economies of scale and achieve better coordination of patient care, a key motivator for the arrangements has undoubtedly been enhanced negotiating leverage with purchasers (Berenson, Ginsburg, Christianson, & Yee, 2012). Indeed, the performance of the many integrated arrangements that were formed during the 1990s was mostly disappointing (Burns & Pauly, 1999). At the same time, provider consolidation has been identified as a key factor in healthcare cost inflation during that same time period (e.g., Vogt & Town, 2006).

More recently, however, new types of delivery models have been advanced that hold promise for improving the quality and efficiency of patient care. Two such models in particular are accountable care organizations (ACOs) and patient-centered medical homes (PCMHs), both of which are generally intended to enhance provider accountability for patient outcomes as well as a focus on patient preferences and needs. In general, ACOs entail a group of providers who jointly assume financial and clinical responsibility for a defined population of patients. As such, ACOs provide largely comprehensive clinical services for patients so that multiple types of professionals and organizations must be integrated, structurally or financially, as part of the arrangement. The PPACA embraced the ACO concept through the creation of several programs that contract with ACOs for assuming responsibility for the care of Medicare enrollees. Many private health insurance plans are also contracting with ACOs or similar types of organizational arrangements for providing care to enrollees (DeVore & Champion, 2011; Higgins, Stewart, Dawson, & Bocchino, 2011; Fisher et al., 2012).

PCMHs generally are physician-directed practices that are intended to provide coordinated and accessible care to patients (Berenson et al., 2008; Friedberg et al., 2015). Under the PCMH model, providers receive payments, whether through fee-for-service or capitated rates, that are supposed to account for the costs of implementing practice infrastructure that supports coordination and continuity of patient care. Additional payments may also be tied to achievement of efficiency and quality targets. Although the PCMH concept was initially targeted to primary care settings, it has been extended to specialty care services (Butcher, 2012). Numerous public- and private-sector purchasers have implemented PCMH programs. Moreover, PCMHs are used in conjunction with ACOs.

Although the impact of these new delivery models on cost, quality, and access remains to be seen (and results have not been impressive in some cases [Hoff, Weller, & DePuccio, 2012]), their diffusion throughout the US healthcare industry is certainly an important development for the health professions. Optimistically, they offer an organizational foundation for developing greater interdisciplinary collaboration among health professionals that can improve patient care. They are also designed to pay providers for services that health professionals often undertake for patients that historically have fallen outside the scope of traditional reimbursement arrangements.

But challenges also exist. ACOs may become settings where health professionals extend and even amplify long-standing turf battles for control over patients and resources. Within the ACO literature, for example, one sees a line of articles staking out positions for the inclusion and prominent role of certain health professionals within this delivery model (e.g., Smith, Bates, & Bodenheimer, 2013; Dupree et al., 2014). Given the association of bundled or global payment mechanisms with ACOs, issues related to which professional groups are in control of budgets and financial decision-making also loom large. Medical homes may have less input from physicians into their design given external pressures from accrediting agencies to conform. Recent research also raises concerns that both regulatory and financial pressures are forcing these delivery models to conform to a rigid one-size-fits-all manner that constrains health professionals from adopting the types of clinical practices needed to meet the preferences and needs of different patients (e.g., Hoff, 2013a).

A Tilt Toward Patients: Consumer Engagement in Healthcare

The move toward a more "consumer-focused" care delivery system represents a significant shift in US healthcare philosophy. It is being driven by corporate interests as well as patients, making it a combined "strategic action" meant to enhance business goals such as profit and a "social movement" meant to shift people's mindsets about their health and involvement in it. It consists of three related parts: (a) a greater focus on patient-centered care through innovative delivery models, particularly in the primary care sphere; (b) using advances in technology such as electronic health records to create "activated" patients that better understand their own health; and (c) the implementation of retail-based philosophies that seek to create long-term, multifaceted relationships with healthcare patients as "consumers" (Bernstein & Vanderlinde-Kopper, 2008; Hoff, 2013b). The first part involves innovations drawing on more traditional parts of the system, such as the implementation of PCMH care models in primary care, using primary care physician practices as the hub for a larger, integrated network of holistic care for patients. The second and third parts involve traditional players in the system but also new ones, some with little prior healthcare experience, yet seeing opportunity in an industry they view as deficient in providing a responsive and deeply satisfying customer experience.

Patient-centered care is defined as the involvement of patients and their families in key aspects of their care delivery, theoretically producing desirable outcomes such as greater patient/family awareness of diseases and treatments, greater shared decision-making with clinicians, a more holistic view of patients in terms of their health status, and greater accountability from patients in caring for themselves. Greater patient-centered care is realized currently through innovations such as the previously discussed PCMHs (National Committee for Quality Assurance [NCQA], 2015), which aim for higher quality patient care experiences through closer connections between patients and primary care physicians, as well as greater emphasis on care coordination, care management, enhanced access, cultural competence, and population health management, among other things (American Association of Family Physicians, 2015).

Supported by an infusion of funds through the Affordable Care Act (ACA) and health insurers, most primary care practices in the United States have achieved some formally recognized status as medical homes (NCQA, 2015). The PCMH model of care has important implications for health professionals given its emphasis on team-based, collaborative care: shifting of work from physicians to others such as nurses and the need for physicians to rely more on their organizational infrastructure to meet the various requirements of the model (Hoff, 2013a). Although the model has produced mixed results (Hoff, Weller, & DePuccio, 2012), it remains an important representation of greater consumer engagement in healthcare.

Technology is a major source of innovation in healthcare that can produce greater consumer engagement with the system. The most important current example is the widespread implementation of electronic medical record (EMR) systems within healthcare organizations. Driven by funding through the ACA aimed at establishing "meaningful use" standards as a common starting point for providers using this technology, EMRs as a harbinger of the larger "e-health" trend have the potential to serve as a vehicle through which provider–patient communication is enhanced; patients are brought closer to managing their own healthcare; various healthcare populations can be segmented and targeted more precisely with appropriate services; and portable, real-time, and up-to-date patient information is made available to those stakeholders in the system who require it most (Detmer, Bloomrosen, Raymond, & Tang, 2008).

The use of EMR systems has implications for how physicians and other health professionals conduct their work, their ability to collaborate, and their interactions with patients. These systems also have implications for how professionals relate to their employers and structure their jobs, including their ability to make decisions and work autonomously. As previously mentioned, EMRs are a form of technology that is being used to standardize the delivery of patient care. However, early research shows large levels of professional frustration with EMR technology, resistance to using it in a fully functional manner, and meaningful impacts in terms of how physicians and patients interact with each other (Miller & Sim, 2004; Boonstra & Broekhuis, 2010). Various issues identified include the misalignment between EMR design and professional workflows, the time commitments required to use EMRs in organizationally desired ways, and the lack of adequate buy-in by professionals to the idea that information technology is a critical innovation to improving care quality.

Other forms of technology such as mobile health (mHealth) applications also may slowly transform how health professionals deliver care and interact with patients. The first-generation mHealth products include wearable devices such as Fitbits and are designed to bring patients into closer, real-time contact with various aspects of their health and diseases. This is accomplished through the monitoring, recording, and transferring of biometric information from patient to physician and medical office. Thus, for example, diabetic patients who require blood glucose checks could use such a device to record their glucose levels and communicate them back in real time to their physicians. Other patients might record weight, caloric intake, and blood pressure, and this information could also be routed back to their physicians on a regular basis.

This information will also then be used directly by patients to self-manage their care. For health professionals, this technology creates new demands and expectations around their interactions with patients. It could fundamentally change the nature of some of their work as well—shifting the model of care from one of reactive response to acute illness to prevention and patient risk management. Among other things, there are important implications for professional time, control, workload, competency development, and job satisfaction from greater use of mHealth technology within healthcare.

Finally, the most profound consumer engagement trend involves the introduction of retail-oriented philosophies and approaches into the US healthcare marketplace (Bernstein & Vanderlinde-Kopper, 2008). The retail philosophy in healthcare involves pursuing several core goals such as treating patients as informed consumers who make careful decisions regarding their healthcare purchases; using segmentation strategies and data analytics to define and target a range of diverse customer needs; and stressing the "four p's" of product, price, promotion, and place in all service delivery. The retail approach is already finding its way into US primary care delivery, through the introduction of retail clinics operated by chains such as CVS and Walmart that stress simplicity, access, price, and convenience in providing medical services to patients. Currently, there are more than 1,800 retail clinics in the United States, accounting for 10 million patient visits annually (Japsen, 2015). This number is expected to grow significantly over the next decade as an aging population and access issues from the additional millions of insured citizens strain the existing primary care system and spur the growth of lower-cost, less physician-centric primary care delivery in rural and inner-city America.

In addition, the ACA and health insurance expansion have created a "direct-to-consumer" insurance marketplace through new public and private exchanges that seeks to provide individuals with greater choice, price transparency, and responsiveness related to the purchase of health insurance coverage (Mercer, 2015). Many of the private health insurance exchanges will evolve to provide "one-stop shopping" to healthcare consumers for services ranging from the related (e.g., access to wellness programs, other healthcare resources) to the unrelated (e.g., other types of insurance, financial services). With its sharp focus on providing an enhanced customer experience through greater engagement between buyer and seller, the retail movement in healthcare should require health professionals such as physicians and nurses to rethink important aspects of how they interact with patients. It also may require health professionals to develop new mindsets and competencies that facilitate treating patients as informed, inquisitive partners in their own care. Certainly, many of the organizations in which these health professionals work, such as hospitals and large practice organizations, will center at least some of their corporate strategy on pursuing the retail approach. Insurance plans that reimburse for provider services are also very interested in using this approach to solidify their relationships with customers.

New and Contested Work Domains Among Health Professionals

Given the increasing pressures related to improving healthcare access and efficiency, a number of professional work domains in US healthcare are increasingly being contested. These contests are facilitated by disruptive innovations such as retail clinics that seek to substitute lower-cost forms of labor to deliver lower-priced, more convenient care to a wider range of individuals. They are also furthered by physician shortages in parts of the country, particularly rural areas, where patient demand is growing due to the expansion of health insurance under the ACA. According to the Health Resources and Services Administration (2015), for example, there are more than 6,000 designated Health Professional Shortage Areas for primary care physicians in the United States. At a macro level, the battle over work jurisdictions in specific areas of healthcare such as primary care creates intraprofessional conflict and competition.

Perhaps the most significant trend in this regard is the expansion of nursing scope of practice laws in many states across the country (Health Affairs, 2013). Twenty-one states now allow nurse practitioners "full practice" autonomy, meaning the ability to "evaluate patients, diagnose, order and interpret diagnostic tests, initiate and manage treatments—including prescribing medications—under the exclusive licensure authority of the state board of nursing" (American Association of Nurse Practitioners [AANP], 2015). Nineteen other states allow nurse practitioners "reduced practice," which means the ability to engage in at least one of the above elements of practice independent of physician oversight (AANP, 2015). Many of the states allowing full practice are located in areas of the country that have significant rural populations and where primary care access is more limited.

Within primary care generally, increased patient demand and primary care physician shortages create imperatives around access that demand the use of innovative models of care delivery; this transfers work duties across professionals and creates new work and roles for physicians, nurses, physician assistants, and pharmacists. These trends are facilitated by healthcare organizations interested in using "physician substitution" approaches to staffing that place intermediaries between physician and patient (Lemieux-Charles & McGuire, 2006). One specific example of this is the move to team care in primary care medicine, particularly concerning chronic disease management. Team care, by often lessening direct contact between physician and patient and replacing it with greater contact between another professional and patient, creates new interprofessional dynamics within healthcare organizations; emboldens professionals other than physicians to seek greater work autonomy; and enhances the legitimacy of these nonphysician groups in the eyes of patients, insurers, and the employing organizations. It also may produce shifting allegiances on the part of patients toward nonphysician personnel within the delivery setting.

The results of such jurisdictional shifts are not all negative. For example, the move to team-based care that uses an array of professional and paraprofessional labor may improve the work cultures within healthcare delivery settings and create a unified, collaborative vision for patient engagement (Lemieux-Charles & McGuire, 2006). It may also lead to greater intraprofessional cooperation and satisfaction among different professional workers. Finally, the interests of physicians and nurses, in particular, coalesce to the extent both groups are similarly employed; required to work together in formal team arrangements; and face identical work- and job-related pressures around time, resources, and performance expectations. In this way, enhanced solidarity may result across these groups vis-à-vis employing organizations, patients, and insurers. As interests converge, the levels of interprofessional trust increase and the levels of conflict may decrease. Health professions traditionally in conflict may grow in solidarity. Among other things, these outcomes will help to redefine how patient care is conducted.

Internal jurisdictional struggles are occurring not just across but within health professions such as medicine and nursing. Because of this, neither of these professions should be considered internally cohesive. For example, within the medical profession, primary care physicians are increasingly ceding their more complex work to various specialties such as cardiology, orthopedics, dermatology, endocrinology, and hospitalists (Hoff, 2010). The drive to squeeze greater efficiencies out of primary care medicine, the increasingly complex nature of some patients' diseases and co-morbidities, and the economics of primary care reimbursement have created a supportive environment for new specialties such as hospital medicine to arise, and for other specialties to lay claim to, select aspects of what traditionally was thought of as within the purview of the primary care physician. This creates tensions and divisiveness within that profession. It also affects the individuals within certain specialties by creating more negative stereotypes around their work and careers. For example, primary care physicians express resentment at the notion that their field is perceived by some medical students as a "consolation prize" to enter into only if other specialties are not attainable (Hoff, 2010).

Within the field of nursing, there are turf battles resulting from the profession's "upskilling" movement (Institute of Medicine, 2010). At a strategic level, this is intended to produce better educated nurses who can fill service gaps in primary care nationally, but it also advances the collective prestige and autonomy of nursing as a whole within healthcare. As nursing seeks to create greater legitimacy for its nurse practitioner professionals, it advances an agenda that may negatively influence lesser skilled nursing positions such as that of licensed practice nurses, for example, in pushing more of its members to gain bachelor's and advanced degrees.

In this vein, the number of nurse practitioners in the United States is expected to double by 2025 (Auerbach, 2012), creating a profession that increasingly will consist of higher paid, more autonomous workers juxtaposed against lower paid, less skilled ones. In addition, the number of nurses holding bachelor degrees has increased to 55% (Health Resources and Services Administration, 2013). Within nursing, this means a more internally stratified membership based on level of education and career expectations. This could translate into fewer collective interests; higher degrees of intraprofessional conflict; and greater heterogeneity related to pay, educational attainment, the socioeconomic backgrounds of members, job conditions, and levels of job and career satisfaction.

The Rise of Expert Consultants Who Shape Health Policy and Management

Additional forces driving change in the health professional workforce include the activities of nongovernmental organizations (NGOs; e.g., the Institute for Healthcare Improvement), voluntary accreditation and quasi-accreditation bodies (e.g., The Joint Commission and Leapfrog group), and professional service firms (e.g., consulting firms, law firms, market research and advertising firms). What these types of organizations have in common is their aim to sell expertise and customized services to healthcare providers. The mechanisms through which these organizations affect change in the health professions are varied and complex. But their effects are consistent with the outcomes of developments described in other sections in this chapter. Accreditation and quasi-accreditation bodies may directly influence changes to health professions and professional and organizational practices through "voluntary" standards (e.g., use of checklists), certifications (e.g., accreditation), or changes to professional norms, requirements (e.g., use of standardized procedures), and regulations (e.g., sentinel event reporting), NGOs and professional service firms may play more subtle, indirect roles as entities that promote among the public new ways of thinking about what it means to be a health professional (e.g., a collaborator rather than solo practitioner) and what it is that patients should expect from their health professionals in terms of the services provided (e.g., a cocreator of care who interacts continually through electronic means). Through these myriad of ways these entities play a key role in the reformation of professions and professional practice.

More specifically, nongovernmental organizations, which have sometimes arisen from social movements in healthcare around safety and quality (e.g., the National Patient Safety Foundation, the National Quality Forum), have been playing an instrumental role for change within the health professional workforce. The Institute for Healthcare Improvement (IHI), an independent not-for-profit organization, aims to improve healthcare by "motivating and building the will for change, identifying and testing new models of care in partnership with patients and healthcare professionals and seeks to ensure the broadest possible adoption of best practices and innovations" (IHI, 2014). The IHI, officially founded in 1991, began in the late 1980s as part of a National Demonstration Project on Quality Improvement in Healthcare led by Donald Berwick and others. Since then, the IHI has grown from an initial collection of grant-supported programs to a self-sustaining organization with worldwide influence (Crisp, 2010). With its 100,000 (or 5 Million) Lives campaigns, the IHI sought to catalyze changes to professional practice, for example in the form of using standardized protocols that could reduce acute care harm and deaths.

Between 2004 and 2008, more than 4,000 hospitals voluntarily participated and pursued 12 interventions to reduce infections, surgical complications, medication errors, and other forms of unreliable care. Eight states enrolled 100% of their hospitals in the campaign, and 18 states enrolled more than 90% of their hospitals in the campaign. An infrastructure of field offices, mentors, and peer teachers was established to provide support for state and local improvement activities (IHI, 2015). Although the IHI acknowledged difficulties in measuring progress toward preventing 5 million instances of harm, evidence showed actual improvement in patient outcomes such as ventilator-associated pneumonia, central line infections, and pressure ulcers. The full impact of the IHI campaign on the health professions cannot be readily assessed, but certainly it has been influential in terms of elevating health professionals' attention to evidence, measurement, standardization, and cost effectiveness of healthcare (IHI, 2015).

Accrediting bodies have also been playing a more significant and direct role in shaping the health professional landscape. The Joint Commission, the oldest and largest standard-setting and accrediting body in US healthcare, evaluates more than 20,500 healthcare organizations and programs seeking "to continuously improve healthcare for the public, in collaboration with other stakeholders, by evaluating healthcare organizations and inspiring them to excel in providing safe and effective care of the highest quality and value" (The Joint Commission, 2015). The Joint Commission has had a direct effect on professional practice through its standards setting. For example, the goal of the sentinel event policy, established in 1996, required hospitals to investigate the root causes of their serious adverse events. The aim was to not only reduce risk, prevent patient harm, and eliminate such events from recurring, but also improve organizational members' capabilities for learning. The National Committee for Quality Assurance (NCQA) exists now as the preeminent quality oversight organization for ambulatory care delivery in the United States. It manages a variety of quality reporting initiatives and data reporting tools such as the Healthcare Effectiveness Data Information Set and the Patient-Centered Medical Home Accreditation Checklist, both of which are used by public and private payers as a means to hold providers more accountable for care delivery (NCQA, 2015).

Finally, professional service firms, or companies that sell services to organizations in multiple industries (Farkas, 2013), are also playing a role in transforming health professions. Professional service firms include organizations such as consulting firms (e.g., Ernst & Young, McKinsey & Company, Truven Health Analytics), law firms, as well as market research (e.g., Deloitte, Accenture), public relations and advertising firms to name a few. These organizations have access to in-depth cross-industry data that enable them to identify opportunities, innovations, and change orientations toward current practice environments. Because of their unique position in bridging stakeholder groups, they import and export ideas and translate them for local contexts, thereby delineating, diffusing, and integrating new meanings and understandings about professional identities and changing professional roles and responsibilities (Suddaby & Greenwood, 2001). For example, most healthcare organizations routinely conduct safety culture surveys to assess the attitudes of a diverse set of organizational members (physicians, nurses, administrators) about acting with safety in mind, fears about speaking up, morale, collaboration, and burnout. Survey findings are fed back to organizational members with the goal of enhancing the climate, promoting more effective teamwork, and overall building more effective organizational cultures.

Fast Forward Through the Book

The remainder of this book covers various topics that speak to how health professions are undergoing transformation, both as a result of internal and external forces driven by US health system change, shifts in social and political climates, and strategic considerations that individual health professions are making to advance their interests and align with demands being placed on them. Each of the following chapters examines different ways in which the health professions are changing and the implications for research, health policy, and healthcare delivery.

Chapter 2 begins with physicians, still at the center of our healthcare delivery system, and examines the various forms of internal stratification within this profession and its implications for specific care delivery, management, and policy issues. Chapter 3 moves to an increasingly important set of other health professions, namely, nurses, pharmacists, and physician assistants—examining the trajectories over time of their roles and training and analyzing how these roles continue to expand, with a synopsis of what it all means for studying and understanding these expert workers.

Chapter 4 considers the very important dynamic of how relationships between healthcare delivery organizations and health professions are changing and the types of governance and decision-making models that are likely to be most effective for building symbiotic working relationships between these two parties. Chapter 5 focuses on the critical ways we must now think about leading and managing health professionals in an era where it is essential that health professions collaborate in the delivery of patient care and where challenges to this imperative present themselves daily within healthcare settings.

Chapter 6 shifts the focus onto professional education and training and trends that will be crucial to selecting and producing expert workers who can align with and contribute effectively towards today's system imperatives. The book's final chapter humbly attempts to identify several major themes that emerge from these other chapters, and attempts to elaborate how such thematic perspectives may inform both research and practice. Finally, many chapters are accompanied by a short commentary piece, written by an influential healthcare stakeholder. This piece, which informs health management, policy, or research, seeks to draw out a key insight or two from a chapter's main points. Brief as they are, these commentary pieces inject a dose of realism into the reader "takeaways" from a chapter, asking readers to consider the analysis presented in specific ways conducive to further dialogue and development.

In its totality, this book is not an exhaustive treatment of the transformations associated with health professions in the United States both now and into the near future. Rather, it offers a critical sampling of key areas of transformation now occurring, and what they may mean for our understanding of how to think about, study, manage, and make policy around these workers. In this sense, the book is less a complete encyclopedia and more a selective anthology. That is, it is meant to generate further discussion and investigations, with the overall aim of creating a more contemporary knowledge base about health professionals working in the United States during the early part of the twenty-first century.

References

American Association of Family Physicians. (2015). *The patient-centered medical home.* Retrieved from: http://www.aafp.org/practice-management/transformation/pcmh.html

American Association of Nurse Practitioners. (2015). *2015 Nurse practitioner state practice environment.* Retrieved from http://www.aanp.org/legislation-regulation/state-legislation-regulation/state-practice-environment

Auerbach, D. L. (2012). Will the NP workforce grow in the future? New forecasts and implications for healthcare delivery. *Medical Care, 50*(7), 606–610.

Baicker, K., Buckles, K. S., & Chandra, A. (2006). Geographic variation in the appropriate use of cesarean delivery. *Health Affairs, 25,* 355–367.

Baker, L. C., Fisher, E. S., & Wennberg, J. E. (2008). Variations in hospital resource use for Medicare and privately insured populations in California. *Health Affairs, 27*(2), 123–134.

Benzer, J., Young, G., Burgess, J., Baker, E., Mohr, D., Charns, M., & Kaboli, P. (2014). Sustainability of quality improvement following removal of pay-for-performance incentives. *Journal of General Internal Medicine, 29*(1), 127–132.

Berenson, R. A., Ginsburg, P. G., Christianson, J. A., & Yee, T. (2012). The growing power of some providers to win steep payment increases from insurers suggests policy remedies may be needed. *Health Affairs, 31*(5), 973–981.

Berenson, R. A., Hammons, T., Gans, D. N., Zuckerman, S., Merrell, K., Underwood, W. S., & Williams, A. F. (2008). A house it not a home: Keeping patients at the center of practice redesign. *Health Affairs, 27*(5), 1219–1230.

Bernstein, A., & Vanderlinde-Kopper, C. (Eds). (2008). *Health care's retail solution: A consumer focused cure for the industry.* Retrieved from http://www.strategyand.pwc.com/media/file/Health_Cares_Retail_Solution.pdf

Birkmeyer, J. D., Sharp, S. M., Finlayson, S. R., Fisher, E. S., & Wennberg, J. E. (1998). Variation profiles of common surgical procedures. *Surgery, 124*, 917–923.

Boonstra, A., & Broekhuis, M. (2010). Barriers to the acceptance of electronic medical records by physicians from systematic review to taxonomy and interventions. *BMC Health Services Research, 10*, 231–248.

Buchman, T. G., Patel, V. L., Dushoff, J., Ehrlich, P. R., Feldman, M., Feldman M, . . . Fitzpatrick, S. (2006). Enhancing the use of clinical guidelines: A social norms perspective. *Journal of the American College of Surgeons, 202*(5), 826–836.

Buntin, M. B., Burke, M. F., Hoaglin, M. C., & Blumenthal, D. (2011). The benefits of health information technology: A review of the recent literature shows predominantly positive results. *Health Affairs, 30*(3), 464–471.

Burwell, S. M. (2015). Setting value-based payment goals—HHS efforts to improve US health care. *New England Journal of Medicine, 372*(10), 897–899.

Butcher, L. (2012). Inside look: First oncology medical home. *Oncology Times, 34*(8), 10.

Cabana, M. D., Rand, C. S., Power, N. R., Wu, A. W., Wilson, M. H., Abboud, P. A., & Rubin, H. R. (1999). Why don't physicians follow clinical practice guidelines? A framework for improvement. *The Journal of the American Medical Association, 282*(15), 1458–1465.

Cima, R. R., Brown, M. J., Hebl, J. R., Moore, R., Rogers, J. C., Kollengode, A., . . . Deschamps, C. (2011). Use of lean and six sigma methodology to improve operating room efficiency in a high-volume tertiary-care academic medical center. *Journal of the American College of Surgeons, 213*(1), 83–92.

Christianson, J. B., Leatherman S., & Sutherland, K. (2008). Lessons from evaluations of purchaser pay-for-performance programs: A review of the evidence. *Medical Care Research and Review, 65*(6), 5S–35S.

Conrad, D. A., & Perry L. (2009). Quality-based financial incentives in health care: Can we improve quality by paying for it? *The Annual Review of Public Health, 30*, 357–371.

Crisp, N. (2010). *Turning the world upside down: The search for global health in the 21st century.* London, UK: CRC Press.

Delbanco, S. (2014). The payment reform landscape: value-oriented payment jumps, and yet . . . *Health Affairs Blog.* September 30. Retrieved from http://healthaffairs.org/blog/2014/09/30/the-payment-reform-landscape-value-oriented-payment-jumps-and-yet/

DeVore, S., & Champion, R. W. (2011). Driving population health through accountable care organizations. *Health Affairs, 30*(1), 41–50.

Dubois, R. W., Batchlor, E., & Wade, S. (2002). Geographic variation in the use of medications: is uniformity good news or bad? *Health Affairs, 21*(1), 240–250.

Dupree, J. M., Patel, K., Singer, S., West, M., Wang, R., Zinner, M., & Weissman, J. (2014). Attention to surgeons and surgical care is largely missing from early Medicare Accountable Care Organizations, *Health Affairs, 33*(6), 972–979.

Eslami, S., Abu-Hanna, A., & de Keizer, N. F. (2007). Evaluation of outpatient computerized physician medication order entry systems: A systematic review. *Journal of the American Medical Informatics Association, 14*(4), 400–406.

Farkas, M. (2013). *Constructing cleantech: The role of sense-giving in the formation of fields.* Doctoral dissertation, University of Michigan.

Fisher, E. S., Shortell, S. M., Kreindler, S. A., Van Critters, A. D., & Larson, B. K. (2012). A framework for evaluating the formation, implementation, and performance of Accountable Care Organizations. *Health Affairs, 31*(11), 2368–2378.

Friedberg, M. W., Chen, P. G., White, C., Jung, O., Raaen, L., . . . Lipinski L. (2015). *Effects of health care payment models on physician practice in the United States.* Retrieved from http://www.rand. org/content/dam/rand/pubs/research_reports/RR800/RR869/RAND_RR869.pdf

Grossman, J. M., Gerland, A., Reed, M. C., & Fahlman, C. (2007). Physicians' experiences using commercial e-prescribing systems. *Health Affairs, 26*(3), 393–404.

Health Affairs. (2013). *Nurse practitioners and primary care.* Retrieved from http://www. healthaffairs.org/healthpolicybriefs/brief.php?brief_id=92

Health Resources and Services Administration. (2013). *The U.S. nursing workforce: Trends in supply and education.* Retrieved from http://bhpr.hrsa.gov/healthworkforce/supplydemand/ nursing/nursingworkforce/nursingworkforcefullreport.pdf

Health Resources and Services Administration. (2015). *Shortage areas, HRSA data warehouse.* Retrieved from http://datawarehouse.hrsa.gov/Topics/ShortageAreas.aspx

Higgins, A., Stewart, K., Dawson, K., & Bocchino, C. (2011). Early lessons from accountable care models in the private sector: Partnerships between health plans and providers. *Health Affairs, 30*(9), 1718–1727.

Hoff, T. (2010). *Practice under pressure: Primary care physicians and their medicine in the 21st century.* Piscataway, NJ: Rutgers University Press.

Hoff, T. (2013a). Medical home implementation: A sensemaking taxonomy of hard and soft practices. *Milbank Quarterly, 91*(4), 771–810.

Hoff, T. (2013b). Towards a diversified future for U.S. Primary care. *American Journal of Managed Care, 19*(1), e9–e13.

Hoff, T., Weller, W., & DePuccio, M. (2012). The patient-centered medical home: A review of recent research. *Medical Care Research and Review, 69*(6), 619–644.

Institute of Medicine. (2010). *The future of nursing: Leading change, advancing health.* Washington, D.C.: National Academy Press.

Institute of Medicine. (2013). *Variation in health care spending: Target decision making, not geography.* Retrieved from http://www.iom.edu/Reports/2013/Variation-in-Health-Care-Spending-Target-Decision-Making-Not-Geography.aspx

Institute for Healthcare Improvement (IHI). (2014). *Financial statements.* Retrieved from http://www.ihi.org/about/Documents/IHIFY2014FinancialStatement.pdf

IHI (2015). Overview of the 100,000 lives campaign. Retrieved from http://www.ihi.org/ Engage/Initiatives/Completed/5MillionLivesCampaign/Documents/Overview%20of%20 the%20100K%20Campaign.pdf

Japsen, B. (2015). Retail clinics hit 10 million annual visits but just 2% of primary care market. Retrieved from http://www.forbes.com/sites/brucejapsen/2015/04/23/retail-clinics-hit-10-million-annual-visits-but-just-2-of-primary-care-market/#4b291523891

The Joint Commission, (2015). About The Joint Commission. Retrieved from http://www.joint-commission.org/

Lemieux-Charles, L., & McGuire, W. L. (2006). What do we know about healthcare team effectiveness: A review of the literature. *Medical Care Research Review*, 63(3), 263–300.

Levay, C., & Waks, C. (2009). Professions and the pursuit of transparency in healthcare: Two cases of soft autonomy. *Organization Studies*, 30(05), 509–527.

Marmor, T. R., & Gordon, R. W. (2014). Commercial pressures on professionalism in American Medical Care: From medicine to the Affordable Care Act. *Journal of Law, Medicine & Ethics*, 42(2), 412–419.

Mercer Marketplace. (2015). Retrieved from http://www.mercer.com/what-we-do/health-and-benefits/private-health-exchange.html

Metzger, J., Welebob, E., Bates, D. W., Lipsitz, S., & Classen, D. C. (2010). Mixed results in the safety performance of computerized physician order entry. *Health Affairs*, 29(4), 655–663.

Mitka, M. (2009). Joint Commission offers warnings, advice on adopting new health care IT systems. *Journal of the American Medical Association*, 301(6), 587–589.

National Committee for Quality Assurance (NCQA). (2015). *Patient-centered medical home recognition*. Retrieved from http://www.ncqa.org/Programs/Recognition/Practices/PatientCenteredMedicalHomePCMH.aspx.

National Center for Health Workforce Analysis, Health Resources and Services Administration. (2013). *The U.S. health workforce chart book*. Retrieved from http://bhpr.hrsa.gov/health-workforce/supplydemand/usworkforce/chartbook/chartbookbrief.pdf

Petersen, L. A., Simpson, K., Pietz, K., Urech, T. H., Hysong, S. J., Profit, J., . . . Woodard, L. D. (2013). Effects of individual physician-level and practice-level financial incentives on hypertension care: A randomized trial. *Journal of the American Medical Association*, 310(10), 1042–1050.

Smith, M., Bates, D. W., & Bodenheimer, T. S. (2013). Pharmacists belong in accountable care organizations and integrated care teams. *Health Affairs*, 32(11), 1963–1970.

Sollecito, W. A., & Johnson, J. K. (2011). *Continuous quality improvement in health care*. Sudbury, MA: Jones and Bartlett.

Suddaby, R., & Greenwood, R. (2001). Colonizing knowledge: Commodification as a dynamic of jurisdictional expansion in professional service firms. *Human Relations*, 54, 933.

Timmermans, S. (2005). From autonomy to accountability. *Perspectives in Biology and Medicine*, 45(4), 490–501.

Van Herck, P., De Smedt, D., Annemans, L., Remmen, R., Rosenthal, M. B, & Sermeus, W. (2010). Systematic review: Effects, design choices, and context of pay-for-performance in health care. *BMC Health Services Research*, 10(247), 1–13.

Vogt, W., & Town, R. (2006). How has hospital consolidation affected the price and quality of hospital care? *Robert Wood Johnson Foundation* Retrieved from http://www.rwjf.org/en/library/research/2006/02/how-has-hospital-consolidation-affected-the-price-and-quality-of.html

Weinstein, J. K., Bronner, K. K., Morgan, T. S., & Wennberg, J. E. (2004). Trends in geographic variations in major surgery for degenerative diseases of the hip, knee and spine. *Health Affairs*, October 7, 81–89.

Westphal, J. D., Gulati, R., & Shortell, S. M. (1997). Customization or conformity? An institutional and network perspective on the content and consequences of TQM adoption. *Administrative Science Quarterly, 42,* 366–394.

Young, G. (2013). Redefining payer-provider relationships in an era of pay-for-performance: A social capital perspective. *Quality Management in Health Care, 22*(3), 187–198.

Young, G., Beckman, H., & Baker, E. (2012). Financial incentives, professional values and performance: A study of pay-for-performance in a professional organization. *Journal of Organizational Behavior, 33,* 964–983.

Young, G., Charns, M., & Shortell, S. (2001). Top manager and network effects on the adoption of innovative management practices: A study of TQM in a public hospital system. *Strategic Management Journal, 22,* 935–951.

2

NOT YOUR PARENT'S PROFESSION

The Restratification of Medicine in the United States

Timothy J. Hoff and Henry Pohl

Introduction

The focus on stratification within medicine is important for several reasons. First, it implies that an increasingly diverse set of interests, needs, expectations, and everyday work realities exist among physician groups that may have an impact on patient care, the profession's status, and organizational relationships. For example, if younger physicians are more interested than their older counterparts in medicine as a "9 to 5 job" and a meaningful work–life balance, the two cohorts may diverge substantially regarding acceptable employment terms, commitment level to patients, and the manner in which particular professional interests are held and advocated for vis-à-vis the larger health system. A highly stratified US medical profession must be understood clearly so that we may in part better predict when that profession may speak and act with one voice, and in which situations it may speak in multiple voices, potentially affecting its overall power and control over select areas of management and policy.

Make no mistake—this is not your parent's medical profession. This is the key takeaway of the chapter. Like other professions such as law, US medicine has been moving from a fairly homogeneous (i.e., in terms of values, demographic makeup, work locations, career choices) collective to a fragmented, sometimes divisive and heterogeneous occupational entity whose primary glue remains the general performance of clinical work and patient care, although that work and care look vastly different from specialty to specialty. For example, primary care physicians have less in common with surgeons and specialists such as cardiologists than ever before and, indeed, often find themselves at odds with specialists over reimbursement, scope of work, and views on how to fix healthcare.

The transformational changes discussed in this chapter cover important demographic shifts within the profession; increased internal fragmentation based on the kinds of clinical work in which physicians engage; new work roles and responsibilities that many physicians face as a result of new career opportunities available to them; innovations such as team-based care; consumer engagement; and the transitioning to a highly corporatized, tightly measured clinical workplace. Physicians have not driven many of these innovations. Rather, they have been pushed on them by managerial forces, policymakers, and outside interests, such as professional service firms (e.g., software vendors) and accreditation and quality assurance organizations, all which have parochial interests to pursue (e.g., profit, cost control, greater operational efficiency) within a transforming US health system now sympathetic to their desires (Hoff, 2010).

Why does an analysis of physician stratification lead a book on transformations in the health professional workforce? There are several reasons.

First, American healthcare has built itself structurally around physicians, in part because it is these professionals who have had the most power to determine how our health system looks. For instance, their embrace of a private insurance model of care, their support for large government programs such as Medicare that pay them well for providing specialty care, their traditional control over when and where high-tech, high-cost medicine is used, and their decades-long advocacy for an acute care model of service delivery are proactive behaviors that have produced a delivery system that reflects their interests and values and, more importantly, makes them the primary focal point of patient trust. The legitimate and referent forms of power accorded to the US medical profession, despite the increasing corporatization of our system, justifies a discussion of this powerful occupational group first.

Second, for better or worse, physicians remain the central decision makers in US healthcare—relating to prescribing, diagnosing, and treating. This role is reinforced by law. They control a good chunk of the healthcare spending in this country; retain the most legitimacy in the eyes of stakeholders such as patients and insurance plans; and have the most say in directing how clinical work is organized, flows, and to what extent others can participate in that process. We can debate whether or not that reality is appropriate, but in the meantime, it exists for the foreseeable future.

Third, many of the other changes occurring to and within health professions such as nursing and pharmacy are significantly influenced by how the changes affecting the medical profession play out. For instance, if younger physicians are more amenable to sharing responsibility for patient care with nurse practitioners (NPs) and physician assistants (PAs), in part because they may place greater emphasis on work–life balance compared to older physicians, then NPs and PAs will find it easier to gain increased autonomy in the workplace and see themselves more legitimized with patients in the process. After all, resistance from physicians is a major reason such groups have been held back from gaining additional independence in their work. But physicians who see NPs and PAs as allies in their quest to remain the types of professionals and workers they wish to be may support these expanded roles.

Finally, there is arguably no other US healthcare workforce component with more change happening in it and to it than physicians. Over the past several decades, US physicians have endured more internal stratification on bases such as age, gender, and specialization than any other healthcare occupation. The work and expectations associated with their roles are also arguably being transformed on a greater scale than NPs and other nurses, pharmacists, PAs, or others in the healthcare sphere. For instance, they never had to think about practicing within a collaborative team structure. Now they increasingly must. Their behavior and decision-making was rarely questioned or monitored. Now there are systems and data in place for just those purposes. Their traditional model of work was face-to-face visits, reimbursed through a fee-for-service schedule dictated by them. Now they are being asked to work within global budgets prospectively given to them, parse out parts of their patient interactions to other personnel to perform, and use technology to deliver "real-time" guidance and instructions to patients. In short, there is more, perhaps substantially more, workforce transformation occurring with US physicians than with anyone else, and so for a book on changes in the health professions workforce, it is important and instructive to lead with some of their unique story.

External Forces Driving Change in the Medical Profession in the United States

The context surrounding doctors within the United States has changed significantly over the past several decades. Much of this change is captured appropriately in other works, and in the introductory chapter of this book. Thus, we will only briefly mention a few key drivers here: (a) societal shifts that place women at the center of a new professional workforce; (b) changes in physician employment relationships; (c) significant outmigration of older physicians out of active practice; (d) increased medical consumption in all facets of US healthcare over the past several decades; (e) a consumer engagement movement in US healthcare that pressures physicians to assume new roles and responsibilities; and (f) the continued corporatization of

US healthcare, including an increased administrative burden associated with managing financial risk and quality in the US healthcare system post–Affordable Care Act (ACA).

INCREASED WORKFORCE DIVERSITY: GENDER, AGE, AND EMPLOYMENT STATUS

The increased presence of women overall in the US workforce over the past several decades, perhaps the most profound stratification trend, is a result of shifts in societal norms as well as the economic realities of lower- and middle-class households. The collective push to establish equality for women in all areas of society has enabled women to enter the workforce in ever greater numbers. In addition, economic realities involving increased family debt and the higher cost of living involved in owning a house, for example, have made it more of an imperative that both parents in a household work. The statistics are telling in this regard. In 1970, women were 38% of the total civilian labor force. In 2012, this same value was 47%—or an increase of approximately 41 million individuals (US Bureau of Labor Statistics, 2014b). Whereas approximately 35% of women with children younger than 3 years of age worked outside the home in 1976, that percentage was 60% in 2012 (US Department of Labor, 2015). Almost 40% of women 25 years of age and older who were working in 2013 had a bachelor's degree or higher, compared to 11% in 1970. This translates into significantly higher percentages of women working in professional fields such as engineering, architecture, law, education, accounting, finance, and medicine (US Bureau of Labor Statistics, 2014b).

With respect to physician employment relationships, physicians are consolidating into larger groups, whether those groups are owned by hospitals, integrated delivery systems, or other physicians. In the early 1980s, 40% of physicians were in solo practice compared to 18% in 2012, and this trend is accelerating (American Medical Association [AMA], 2013). The majority of physicians still work in smaller practices (e.g., fewer than 10 physicians) but increasingly as salaried employees rather than equity owners (AMA, 2013). Two factors underlie this trend.

First, both the scale and financial resources needed to operate a viable physician practice have increased substantially, forcing physicians to ally themselves with larger, resource-rich organizations such as hospitals and physician "supergroups." Also, organizations such as hospitals place enhanced value on putting physicians on the payroll, given the reimbursement trends associated with the ACA (Jackson Healthcare, 2013; Physicians Foundation, 2010). Physicians working as employees for these organizations often cite the "administrative hassles" and "business pressures" of the present healthcare system that drive them into salaried work (Jackson Healthcare, 2013).

Second, age-based demographic shifts are occurring in US medicine. This involves the outmigration of a large cohort of physicians in the United States older than the age of 55, many of whom were reared during a time when owning one's practice was both normal and made financial sense. As they begin to work part-time and retire in greater numbers, they are being replaced by younger physicians with a greater willingness to work as salaried employees and for large healthcare organizations, in part because of the large debt loads carried from medical school, which produces the risk aversion to investing in one's own practice. In 2012, the median education debt for students attending medical schools within the United States was $160,000 for public schools and $190,000 for private schools (American Association of Medical Colleges [AAMC], 2012). Annual median education debt for US medical school graduates has increased 6.3% per year since 1992, well above the normal annual rate of inflation for the same time period (AAMC, 2012).

These two factors, coupled with a desire among young physicians to pursue a more balanced lifestyle than many of their predecessors (Dorsey, Jarjoura, & Rutecki, 2003), including a greater emphasis on nonwork roles, makes physician ownership of medical practices less likely moving into the future. The value systems of the millennial generation differ greatly from that of both baby boomers and generation Xers, and these differences create divergent perceptions of medicine as a profession (Drake, 2014). One of these perceptions is of medicine more as a "good job" rather than "all-encompassing calling" (Hoff, 2010).

Younger physicians remain more optimistic about the current direction of US healthcare than their older colleagues (Physicians Foundation, 2012). This is true despite their greater tendency to work as salaried employees and not as owners of their own practices. This optimism includes more positive feelings about the state of the US medical profession, higher personal morale, less negative perceptions about being employed by organizations such as hospitals, greater embrace of health information technology, and a greater belief in the transformative potential of structural innovations such as accountable care organizations and patient-centered medical homes (Physicians Foundation, pp. 63–78). Whether or not these differences shape various patient and physician outcomes differently is an empirical question. But what remains clear is that younger physicians over time will contribute to important shifts in the professional workplace.

CHANGES ON THE DEMAND SIDE: MEDICAL CONSUMPTION AND CONSUMER ENGAGEMENT

The increased societal preference for medical consumption as a result of liberal insurance policies for many middle-class workers through the 1960s, 1970s, and 1980s, as well as the ultimate rejection of managed care principles in the 1990s that sought to rein in both unfettered choice and healthcare costs, have produced within US medicine a hyperspecialization trend. This has been facilitated by advances in clinical science and medical technology. This trend has greatly wounded primary care and the system's emphasis on prevention and keeping people healthy. The nation's love affair with high-tech medicine and with specialist physicians will not end any time soon. The US population is aging fast, creating a larger group of patients who arguably require specialty care because of the presence of more chronic diseases. In addition, the decline of primary care and a healthcare system philosophy of treating most people after they are already sick, along with poorer eating habits and unhealthier lifestyles among much of our population conspire to fuel the internal divisiveness of a US medical profession now composed of many rival factions and competing financial interests.

It has also produced a medical–industrial complex in which physicians increasingly find themselves subservient, even those from the most prestigious specialties. For example, the rise of a nonclinical managerial class to administer health services delivery in the US enables healthcare organizations such as hospitals to partially wrench control over medical decision making and investment from physicians (US Bureau of Labor Statistics, 2014a). In the 21st century, health services delivery in the United States is a complex, costly endeavor to administer, which fuels the physician employment trend and lends greater credence to the need for a larger administrative structure around physicians' work.

With the advent of the ACA, this complexity will continue, along with downward cost pressures in parts of the industry that will spur consolidation, through new structures such as accountable care organizations. Among other things, these new structures may be able to handle the shared risk necessary for new payment systems that reward outcomes of care. Cost pressures will also spur hospital mergers and acquisitions, which in some geographic areas of the country create monopolistic organizations that seek to gain control over physician networks as feeders for their own services. Mergers and acquisitions among health insurers (Bomey, 2015) also stand to affect professional stratification in medicine as fewer insurance plans may hold greater sway over physicians through the formation of limited provider networks and also by advocating (through paying or not paying for) certain types of physician services over others.

Remaining financially viable as a practicing physician in today's US health system requires enough capital and managerial awareness to invest in personnel such as care coordinators, billing staff, and infrastructure such as sophisticated electronic medical record systems and ancillary services for patients aimed at chronic disease management. In addition, the focus on consumer engagement in healthcare affects how the US medical profession thinks and behaves. For example, patients have moved from being thought of as purely paternalistic recipients of physician wisdom, to more proactive consumers encouraged to ask questions, raise concerns, and take greater accountability for their conditions (Bernstein & Vanderlinde-Kopper, 2008).

Enhanced consumer engagement is supported in meaningful ways by outside (of healthcare) corporate interests looking to create new markets for their products. These products include disruptive innovations such as retail clinics, which offer a relatively low-cost model of basic primary care delivery by placing less emphasis on physicians in favor of less expensive types of providers. The proliferation of mobile health applications and the technology to support them are intended to give patients more control over their health through proactive self-management. In addition, although the "yelpification" of healthcare (Abrams, 2012) still has not occurred on a scale commensurate with enhancing patient power at the expense of physician power, physicians do face increased public scrutiny of their clinical behaviors through various rating and report card efforts led by organizations such as Healthgrades.com, Vitals. com, and Medicare.

Although these efforts are moving slowly due to a variety of factors, they are beginning to create more broad-based support for greater transparency of physician behavior and performance. It is not difficult to imagine that such efforts will only grow in significance as people are able to gather and make sense of more data related to physicians and their work. In addition, as members of the millennial generation advance to and through adulthood, they will expect this type of transparency within medicine as everywhere else, where they function as proactive consumers. This is especially true because this generation's level of trust and attachment to traditional societal institutions is much less than the generations before them (Drake, 2014). US medicine could conceivably move to a more heavily retail-oriented model of service delivery: a model in which patients as "consumers" are segmented into different subgroups based on the desire to create and sell a host of health and non–health-related products to them (Deloitte Center for Health Solutions, 2012). The greater placement of healthcare corporations as intermediaries between physicians and their patients, in the name of product expansion and profit, has the potential to change both the expectations and perceptions the two groups have of each other. It may also pressure physicians to participate more in a wider variety of service provision for patients, even some services that are less directly health-oriented.

Increased Physician Diversity in Medicine in the United States

The forces described above and in Chapter 1 have helped to propel the US medical profession to a state of increased internal diversity along a number of dimensions.

These dimensions include gender, age, clinical specialization, and type of work role. The diversity we see today and in the near future within the US medical profession weakens professional solidarity, creates an internally competitive profession, and cultivates everyday interests and expectations that differ from physician to physician. The question of whether US medicine can speak with one collective voice to important management and policy questions in healthcare today seems already answered: it cannot. What remains now is to understand both the bigger picture implications of a diverse profession and how this diversity shifts workforce priorities related to physicians in ways that merit new ways of thinking.

THE NEW BREED OF PHYSICIAN: DIFFERENT BELIEFS, EXPERIENCES, NEEDS, AND EXPECTATIONS

Mirroring the larger US workforce, there is no more profound demographic development occurring in US medicine than the increasing number of women who are becoming physicians. Half of all US medical school graduates are now women (AAMC, 2012). In 1965, less than 10% of all US medical school applicants were female. In 2010, that percentage had increased to approximately 50% (AAMC, 2012). Approximately 30% of the active US physician workforce is now female, compared to 7% in 1970. As older male physicians retire in greater numbers, female physicians will become an even larger part of the whole. Female physicians are disproportionately over-represented in primary care specialties and under-represented in surgical subspecialties such as orthopedics, urology, and thoracic surgery (AAMC, 2012).

What is so transformational about a profession with a significant female population? For one, it can shift in key ways the dynamics between organization and physician, physician and physician, physician and patient, and physician and other members of the health team. There is relevant research here, which informs these issues. Female physicians have been shown to practice differently than male physicians. For example, they may communicate differently with patients, focusing more intently on the underlying social-emotional context surrounding illness (Roter, Hall, & Aoki, 2002). They may also spend greater time in the clinical encounter focusing on prevention and counseling patients, rather than on the physical aspects of the interaction such as the clinical examination (Bertakis & Azari, 2003; Hoff, 2010). Female physicians may take more time listening to patients than male physicians (Roter et al., 2002). They also bring different skill sets to the everyday work of medicine; these skill sets may facilitate greater effectiveness as members of clinical teams and working one-on-one with patients (Aruguete & Roberts, 2000).

Female physicians face similar job discrimination and career barriers as their female counterparts in other occupations (Hoff & Scott, 2015). For example, they are often paid less than male physicians, beginning at the very outset of their careers (LoSasso, Richards, Chou, & Gerber, 2011), and this pay inequity persists even when doing the same clinical job (Hoff, 2004; Danesh-Meyer et al., 2007; Jagsi et al., 2012). They face other forms of workplace discrimination, in particular a lack of career advancement opportunities compared to their male counterparts (Kass, Souba, & Thorndyke, 2006; Reed, Enders, Lindor, McClees, & Lindor, 2011; Cochran et al., 2013). Perhaps most importantly, female physicians make many greater trade-offs in their jobs, work, and careers than male physicians, and this reality in part reflects their different set of needs and preferences. Female physicians are more likely than their male counterparts, particular early in their medical careers, to have to work part-time and to be under greater pressure from nonwork roles such as spouse and parent (Hoff, 2010; Hoff & Scott, 2015). They also express greater dissatisfaction with their ability to achieve adequate work–life balance while reporting a greater sacrifice of work and career compared to male physicians (Danesh-Meyer et al., 2007; McAlister, Jin, Braga-Mele, DesMarchais, & Buys, 2014).

Younger physicians, whether male or female, are also poised to transform certain elements of US medicine, largely because their value systems and job expectations differ from their older counterparts. More than one-third of American physicians are older than age 55. These older physicians, who came of age at a time of economic and cultural dominance for the medical profession (Starr, 1982), were trained and socialized to believe being a physician meant having little of an outside life, particularly early in one's career. Instead, this time was to be spent building a dedicated patient base and proving oneself (usually through a display of work ethic that included the total number of hours worked each week) to physician colleagues in order to have the opportunity to buy into ownership in a practice. As these older physicians retire or reduce their work hours, they are replaced by a millennial generation of practitioners who clearly want to work less and put their professional obligations in the context of their total lives, which includes their nonwork roles and activities (AAMC, 2012; Glicksman, 2013). To facilitate these values, younger physicians in the United States are much more comfortable placing greater work responsibility on nonphysician staff, are amenable to using technology to create virtual work spaces, and may be more open to placing greater responsibility on the patient to manage their care (Katz, 2011; Silverman, 2014).

Some older physicians view these values and beliefs in a negative light, for example, as a retreat from the full-fledged professional duties that one accepts when signing on for one of the toughest professions in American work life (Hoff, 2010). Others are more ambivalent, shrugging their shoulders at a generation whose greater tendencies towards non-work pursuits, personal awareness and immediate gratification bleed into every aspect of who they are and what they do (Ng, Schweitzer, & Lyons, 2010). The younger physicians' different outlook and beliefs have implications for the healthcare system and how it interacts with them.

For instance, the particular values and expectations of these physicians make them more amenable to working as salaried employees and for larger organizations that can assume key nonclinical responsibilities for them. The desire to work fewer hours and experience less administrative hassles may be exchanged for a willingness to submit to greater control to the organization, performance measurement systems, and external oversight. It also may make younger physicians a professional audience more likely to comply with organizational edicts around quality and efficiency and new forms of work organization such as clinical teams.

MEDICAL SPECIALIZATION AND THE FRAGMENTED INTERESTS COMPETING IN MEDICINE IN THE UNITED STATES

Another important source of US physician diversity derives from clinical specialization. The Association of American Medical Colleges lists more than 120 medical specialties and subspecialties on its website for new medical residents. The number of specialties has proliferated over the past several decades, spurred by advances in medical science and technology, a sicker general population, organized medicine's collective interest in furthering high-cost care delivery, an emphasis on acute rather than primary care within the system, and the general public's embrace of specialist medicine. These various specialties involve vastly different forms of clinical work, have dedicated insurance reimbursement streams and staff associated with them, and are often practiced within different organizational settings. Although they are all under the banner of the US medical profession, many of these specialties have little in common and, in fact, work at cross-purposes to advance their own interests at the expense of others (Rosenthal, 2014).

A lot is on the line in this high-stakes, intraprofessional competition. As a form of stratification, it has reduced organized medicine in the United States to little more than a loose confederation of independent physician groups—groups of highly educated, well-paid "haves" and "have nots." The first fault line lay in the issue of specialty compensation. The 25 highest-paid specialties have an annual income gap between the highest and lowest paid of $250,000 (Herman, 2013). That said, even dermatologists, who represent the 25th highest-paid specialty, earn approximately $250,000 to $300,000 more annually than pediatricians or family physicians. More than 40 different medical specialties have an individual lobbying presence in Washington, DC, and each of these groups support legislation that is often uniquely beneficial to their specialty but not to others.

The second fault line is found in public perception. Not all US medical specialties are viewed equally in terms of status, knowledge base, skill complexity, and importance. For example, whereas primary care specialties such as family medicine and pediatrics are viewed as central to health and accorded higher status in countries such as the United Kingdom and Canada, such specialties are perceived by many in the United States as involving less skill, fewer "life-and-death" situations, and more "basic" medicine. Such public perception is a reason why primary care medicine in the United States receives lower insurance reimbursements than specialty care, why many patients in the United States seek specialty care on a frequent basis, and why primary care physicians (PCPs) earn less in their jobs relative to other types of physicians. In the United States, specialties such as neurosurgery, cardiology, neurology, and orthopedics receive the most recognition by the general public.

This stratification of specialties by the level of public prestige accorded each produces further tensions and divisiveness within the profession. For example, PCPs, in particular, come to resent the power and privilege, as well as higher compensation, accorded these other specialties (Hoff, 2010). In addition, this can contribute to workplace ambivalence among physicians from different specialties when they are forced to care simultaneously for the same patient. For example, in research performed by one of the authors, feedback from PCPs indicated a high level of care coordination challenges among different types of physicians caring for the same patient, with PCPs believing that they shouldered much of the work and got little cooperation from specialists. This made PCPs feel more resentful toward some of their specialist colleagues, and in some instances this led to avoidance between the groups where greater interaction around patient care was needed (Hoff, 2010). From a workforce perspective, clinical collaboration among different physicians becomes more difficult when perceptions of physician specialties is such that some are viewed as "more skilled" or "higher status" and thus end up in greater demand by patients and compensated better by payers.

THE NEW WORK ROLES AND RESPONSIBILITIES FOR PHYSICIANS IN THE UNITED STATES

The changes occurring in the US healthcare system provide a diverse array of new work and career opportunities for physicians. This represents another form of internal stratification. Traditionally, a physician in the United States had few alternative job choices other than that of being an active clinician. A few became medical directors or chairs of services or departments, but there was little else from which to choose. Physicians moving into executive roles were also viewed in a much more negative light by other colleagues, the latter whom often viewed them as "traitors" to their profession (Hoff, 1999). However, the advent of a more corporatized health system means a wider array of management jobs for physicians, as well as a legitimization of these nonclinical roles. Some of the names of these diverse roles include chair, medical director, consultant, director of medical affairs, clinical team leader, director, and quality improvement manager. A professional association, the American Association of Physician Leadership, has legitimized the physician executive.

The diversity of physician roles continues to increase. For example, increased emphasis on efficiency and quality in US healthcare has created a wide array of physician jobs in areas such as quality management and utilization management. The growing complexity of healthcare reimbursement has also led to new physician careers in areas such as contracting and risk management. Advances in technology and the proliferation of "big data" require physicians willing to assume jobs in population health, public health, chronic disease management, and information management. Finally, increased physician shortages and retention problems across various clinical specialties, as well as the need for healthcare organizations to pursue robust talent management strategies for their physician-employees has created positions in the area of human resources and human resources consulting for physicians, who are often viewed as having a better understanding of needs and preferences their colleagues now possess.

Very often, the types of positions described above are embedded within larger healthcare organizations such as hospitals, integrated delivery systems, independent practice association-type physician practice networks, organizations providing health services (e.g., CVS, Walgreens), consulting groups, and larger multispecialty practices. This puts them squarely into the purview of corporate medicine, and such a reality may further stratify the US medical profession in ways that lead to divergent interests among its members. Closer to the clinical practice level, the proliferation of new models of care delivery also create new types of work and responsibilities for physicians. Team-based care delivery, the use of intermediaries such as healthcare coaches and care navigators, and the expanded use of NPs and PAs to provide direct care has encouraged many physician clinical practices to create formal management positions for physicians that oversee and evaluate these new models of care delivery, or that serve as the de facto leaders of a collaborative approach to health delivery that uses many different types of personnel.

Implications of an Increasingly Diversified Medical Profession in the United States

The types of internal stratification now occurring within the US medical profession has important implications for theory, research, and practice. How we think about physicians, how we try to better understand them as professionals and workers, and the questions we choose to investigate are all informed by better appreciating the diversity now being visited upon this group. To that end, the following section highlights some of these implications.

Physician Identity and Commitment Are Increasingly Diverse, Which Means Behavior is Less Predictable and Loyalties May Be Split. The fragmentation of the US medical profession along the lines of key values, beliefs, preferences, and work experiences has important implications for physician identity and commitment. Physician identity and commitment are important concepts because both shape how these practitioners behave in the workplace. Perhaps the most important of these implications is the emerging reality of work and professional identities that look somewhat different across the various substrata of physicians. The traditional view held that these clinicians pursue a collective form of self-interest that defends and advances purely professional interests, even at the expense of organizational or managerial imperatives (Larson, 1977). This view made physician behavior highly predictable, motivated by values such as autonomy, economic control, the advancement of science, and patient ethics. Jurisdictional battles over aspects of healthcare work were more easily explained through this lens as instances of physicians extending their turf in ways consistent with their perceived right to control a work domain economically, politically, and clinically (Abbott, 1988).

In the modern healthcare workplace, some physicians may still exhibit this "pure" form of professionalism that centers on the control over clinical knowledge and the unfettered application of that knowledge in professional–client interactions (Freidson, 1970). These may be physicians who are still less likely to work as salaried employees. More likely to be high-prestige specialists, they are less comfortable in aligning themselves with organizational imperatives like pay for performance. But many other groups of physicians in the future will exhibit identities and forms of commitment that involve loyalty to multiple targets beyond simply their profession, professional colleagues, and even patients. One increasingly common loyalty target is the organization that employs a given physician. Most physicians in the future will likely work as salaried employees for a larger corporate entity, whether run by other physicians, hospitals, or new structural innovations such as accountable care organizations.

It is the physician's employing organization that will play a significant role in personal career development, financial compensation, job flexibility, and the creation of an everyday workplace that maintains satisfaction and prevents burnout. In return for this involvement in meeting their individual interests, physicians may increasingly commit themselves to the (a) pursuit of corporate or managerial goals such as greater efficiency in delivering care, (b) greater embrace of team work structures, (c) use of technology in their work, and (d) greater transparency related to having their work and decision-making monitored. In some cases, they may be willing to be questioned for the purpose of standardizing some patient care, lowering care costs, and improving quality. In short, both their identities as professionals and work loyalties may grow fragmented, and these loyalties could complement or compete with each other in ways that affect workforce dynamics and care delivery.

Theories of professions generally, and of medicine specifically, are still grappling with how best to conceptualize the identity focus of modern-day physicians. Rather than trying to reconcile this variety through yet another grand theory of "professions," what is required are more "middle-range" concepts and ideas (Merton, 1967) that extend directly from our observed understanding of the forms of stratification described in this chapter. For instance, the more we study how these different forms of stratification shape not only individual identity but also clinical decision-making, patient care, and physician relationships with other occupations, the better able we are to develop new explanatory ideas for how physicians think and behave.

In this way, variables that serve as the basis for modern-day physician stratification such as age and gender must become more than atheoretical controls in empirical work. They should be richly specified explanatory vehicles that predict outcomes such as quality of care, interprofessional relations, job satisfaction, burnout, career and job choices, and innovation adoption. Practically speaking, US physicians must be managed more not as an homogenous group with uniformly predictable thinking and behavior, as they have traditionally been, but instead as diverse groups of talent, whose motivations for thought and action across different work contexts are less overtly known-highly dependent on their everyday context. In addition, whose ability to act in accordance with desired organizational or system goals can be manipulated through policies and incentives that align with their more parochial interests.

Physician Power and Legitimacy Should be Reconsidered and Focused on How Such Dynamics Are Increasingly Negotiated at the Workplace Level. Both physician power and legitimacy vis-à-vis the public, regulators, healthcare organizations, and other healthcare workers must be reconsidered given a US medical profession that is diversified in the ways described above. One reconsideration we already know much about is how the balance of power among clinical specialties within US medicine has shifted over the past several decades. PCPs have acquiesced, whether consciously or not, to the interests of higher-paying procedural specialties, supported by public perceptions that the latter is more prestigious and skilled. This is playing out in the disproportionate power and influence the latter specialties exert at both federal and state policy levels, particularly in controlling reimbursement through mechanisms such as the Relative Value Scale Update Committee, or the RUC, which is a small group of physicians from 29 different medical specialties. The vast majority of these physicians, who are not representatives of primary care, make recommendations to the government about how much different services and procedures should be valued and ultimately reimbursed (Moore, Felger, Larimore, & Mills, 2008).

But there are other newly emerging power and legitimacy dynamics emanating from the stratification trends described. These dynamics will be resolved largely at the workplace level, through the day-to-day negotiations and trade-offs occurring among physicians as they seek to navigate an increasingly complex, uncertain, and in some cases hostile work situation. For example, the influx of women into the profession could raise questions of how medicine's collective power versus other institutions and interests within the healthcare industry is affected, if at all. Historically, occupations with a significant percentage of females are perceived as lower in status and prestige (Murgatroyd, 1982). But given that women are now embedded in large numbers in most every occupation, that traditional view is not as pertinent to understanding how an enhanced female presence in medicine could shape physician power and legitimacy. Instead, it may be more relevant to understand, for example, the real issues of gender inequality within medicine that merit greater study and collective intervention (Hoff & Scott, 2015).

Indeed, it is this inequality that if left unaddressed threatens some of the societal legitimacy accorded physicians, and could weaken the profession's collective ability to influence the direction of healthcare management and policy in the United States. For instance, if healthcare employers are allowed to treat female physicians differently than their male colleagues, and this treatment involves discriminatory practices, pay disparities, or attempts to exact significant concessions from women because of their greater tendency to desire certain job or career arrangements, the US medical profession's collective influence could suffer, as well as the localized control physicians exert over patient care, the terms of their employment, and healthcare decision making.

In short, the profession may cede power and control in key areas to nonprofessional interests or even other healthcare occupations. Equally important, the type of internal conflict such inequities may facilitate, for example, between male and female physicians, and between different clinical specialties that remain slanted toward one gender or the other in terms of membership, could also weaken the profession's ability to speak as a unified voice and to influence key debates related to the health policy issues of the day.

A related issue concerns the different values and preferences of younger physicians, particularly with respect to wanting to work less, working for larger organizations and as salaried employees, and emphasizing nonwork interests. These preferences might reshape public perception of the medical profession. Will these preferences lower the perceived prestige of the profession among the US general public, which has long been used to seeing their physicians as independent experts who work around-the-clock and defend them against other stakeholders such as insurance companies? At a workplace level, will younger physicians be willing to trade traditional professional values such as autonomy, which form the basis for physician hegemony, in return for organizationally controlled rewards such as better work hours, time off, and higher pay?

The embedding of physicians across all specialties within large, corporatized organizational settings, and the growing alignment of younger physicians with these organizations make some aspects of professional power increasingly threatened and consigned to resolution on a case-by-case basis. From a research standpoint, the interesting empirical questions moving forward focus on how the acquisition, maintenance, and exertion of physician power are *negotiated* among individual physicians and their employing organizations, insurers, and other healthcare workers.

This focus has been around for several years. However, it remains mysteriously avoided by many researchers, even as it has implications for key outcomes such as efficiency and care quality. What trade-offs are physicians willing to make with respect to giving up some forms of power and legitimacy, in return for satisfying their other interests? In what work situations will the balance of power and control tip toward individual physicians versus managers, the larger organization, or insurers? Which particular combinations of physician and organizational control within a setting most benefit patients? All of these are questions that must move front-and-center in the study of the US medical profession, and they must be informed by knowledge of the stratification forces now occurring within it.

Practically, the US health system's desire to increase patient engagement and adopt "patient-centric" care models depends meaningfully on physicians' ability to shape key debates around what should be expected of patients, how best to involve them in clinical decision-making, where patient accountability should be tempered, and what roles different types of health professionals should play. Physicians offer a needed counterbalance to other perspectives on how to engage patients, for example, and it is important they have the ability to speak as one within whatever work settings they find themselves. Given the increased consideration to incorporating retail philosophies into healthcare (Bernstein & Vanderlinde-Kopper, 2008) and the shifting of greater financial responsibility onto patients through consumer-directed health plans, strengthening physician solidarity within the workplace, and building influential coalitions among physicians and other health occupations loom as key strategic imperatives in the power negotiation process.

The Talent Management Needs of US Physicians Require Radical Rethinking. The traditional view of US medicine as an internally homogenous profession coupled with the prior reality of many physicians working for themselves or within small physician-owned groups absolved healthcare organizations for a long time from seeing the practitioners as human capital requiring cultivation and maintenance. But US physicians of all types now merit proactive engagement on the human resources front. No longer are the vast majority of physicians coming out of residency looking for the same thing (i.e., a good clinical job, the potential to become part owner of their practice, and a high degree of clinical and economic autonomy).

The cases of younger and female physicians are instructive in this regard. For example, female physicians have been shown to lack appropriate mentoring (Hoff & Scott, 2015). Given some of their unique work circumstances, these clinicians could benefit from role models and career guidance that can help them overcome workplace obstacles to their careers. Younger physicians, male or female, clearly see medicine in a different light than many of their older colleagues, which raises unique talent management needs for this cohort as well. Those needs may include assistance with paying off loans, guidance on how to fulfill the everyday demands of a full-time clinical job within a set amount of weekly hours, long-term career advice and continuing education about managing complex patients, working in a team-based environment, and meeting organizational goals related to quality and efficiency. Organizations that employ large numbers of young or female physicians also must consider that part of their talent management approach for the future is to redesign jobs and workplaces in ways that fit the diverse preferences of these groups. This may include innovative approaches that involve job and patient sharing, as well as conducting patient care virtually and from home. Examining the impact of these new arrangements on outcomes such as physician satisfaction and burnout, as well as on healthcare quality and patient experience, must also be a component of the overall talent management strategy.

Important conceptual development must also occur to explain the (a) various talent management requirements for different groups of physicians and (b) personal and contextual factors that drive these requirements. We need better theories in the area of human resources management with respect to physicians—and perhaps all professionals. Among other things, this requires a greater synthesizing of literatures that rarely speak to each other (i.e., the sociology of professions and the organizational behavior literature). It also requires comparative analysis in which scholars specify how and why physicians are similar or different from other types of healthcare workers.

In addition, research must examine how best to engage physicians in the realm of talent management—that is, how to screen and assess their needs and desires, which types of interventions and services align with their particular needs, and the different ways in which some groups should be approached to ensure the most support for organizational efforts. Organizationally, greater financial investment and time should be placed into the physician talent management endeavor. In this respect, there may be economies of scale that occur through the linking of physician talent management needs related to job and career with similar needs other professionals such as nurses and pharmacists exhibit in these areas. For example, some physicians will benefit from similar types of career development interventions as others, for example, if they are interested in management positions, work in different structures such as teams, or possess similar terms of employment. Similarly, issues related to fair compensation, having a voice in organizational decision-making, and preventing job-related burnout—these are issues physicians as well as other health professionals are increasingly concerned with in their everyday work.

Different Physicians Will Be Used for Different Models of Care. From an applied standpoint, greater intraprofessional diversity within US medicine may benefit patients, especially to the extent that different types of professionals with unique talents, work preferences, and belief systems can be aligned to better fit a range of new care delivery models. Take the example of clinical teams. The most proven predictors of successful team outcomes are what might be termed "relational" aspects of teams that include both social and psychological elements. Examples of these include psychological safety, participation, empowerment, communication, work climate, and role clarity. Within the health services, clinical, and business literatures these "softer" type variables turn up repeatedly as significant drivers of effective team functioning (for a detailed review of the team literature, see Cohen & Bailey, 1997).

The implications of these particular findings for which types of physicians to place into team structures is simple: teams require those physicians who possess personal qualities and work styles that facilitate the above dynamics, especially because the physician is usually viewed as the de facto leader of the team. With an appreciation for medicine's intraprofessional diversity, it becomes clear that not all physicians will perform well in team structures, because not all physicians are effective communicators, have participative work styles, are comfortable interacting as co-equals with their nonphysician colleagues, or want to play a proactive role in being a liaison between what their organization requires and patient expectations.

A key workforce focus in this respect is to find ways, going as far back as medical school, to assess individuals on the basis of key personality traits, leadership profiles, types of professional identities, and work preferences, with the intent to steer them into positions and career tracks where their unique talents and interests can make a bigger contribution. This closer alignment between the these types of physician characteristics and specific job or career placements may also over time lessen some of the intense career regret and job dissatisfaction now existing within US medicine (Physicians Foundation, 2012). However, extending the example, this is not to say that all female physicians will be good at one type of clinical job or care focus or that older physicians should be assigned to more complex care duties than their younger, less experienced colleagues. The stratification occurring within US medicine is neither neat nor clean with respect to identifying large groups of physicians who will uniformly be better suited than others to specific work or employment situations. Rather, the key point is that greater recognition of physician differences inevitably leads to better efforts to understand this diversity and how it may be used strategically to provide better healthcare, more satisfied workers, and effective innovation implementation.

The Assimilation or Transformation Question Must Be Studied Extensively. Other questions loom large in considering the implications of this internal stratification within US medicine. For example, a viable research agenda, with practical implications, can address the general question of whether these demographic groups will ultimately assimilate into the existing profession's norms, values, and belief systems, or instead transform those existing norms, values, and beliefs in ways that ripple through other segments of the profession. Longitudinal study of the assimilation versus transformation question is needed. This should entail tracking changes in the various belief and value systems over time across segments of the profession and connecting them with a variety of outcomes about patient care, professional attitudes and behavior, and implementation dynamics.

Take the case once again of female physicians. Although some early research shows that female physicians bring different qualities and experiences to the practice of medicine, it is fair to ask if these differences remain true as larger numbers of women move further along in their careers and, more importantly, as they move into traditional male-dominated specialties such as surgery in greater numbers, where the peer pressure to perform one's role in a more prescribed (to the traditional norms) manner is greater. To this end, there is evidence that shows that for some female physicians, assimilation into the existing ways of thinking does happen (Marley, Lerner, Panagopoulos, & Kavaler, 2011). If assimilation ends up the primary dynamic, then we may not see a profession that changes all that much in terms of how its members enact their roles on an everyday basis and what larger workforce policies the profession advocates for with employers, payers, and government.

We are not necessarily making normative statements about whether existing physician role enactments, some of which have been the norm for years are good or bad, or in need of modification. Rather, we are suggesting that (a) it is presumptuous to assume that the types of diversity we see occurring in US medicine will naturally lead to profoundly different ways of thinking and acting across the entire profession or (b) its effects are entirely predictable. More than likely, some stratification will yield a transformative effect, whereas others will not. But from both a policy and management perspective, knowing something more about whether or not, for example, the values and role expectations of female physicians will bleed into and affect those of male physicians becomes strategically important. The structure of physician jobs and compensation systems, the talent management foci to adopt, how to match physicians to the most appropriate patient care situations, and developing reimbursement policies that can gain widespread acceptance—these are examples of questions for which a deeper knowledge of the assimilation versus transformation dynamic, across multiple stratification realities, is beneficial.

Conclusion: Physician Stratification and the Healthcare Workforce

Much is changing within the US medical profession. This chapter has sought to outline some of the key stratifying trends now occurring within it; the external and internal forces driving those trends; and the key issues they may have an impact such as professional power and legitimacy, work and career identity, care delivery, and the ways in which healthcare organizations manage physician talent. These are merely a sampling of the larger array of patient care, workforce, and policy issues raised by a US physician workforce that continues to undergo meaningful change. In particular, it is relevant to ask what this workforce will look like a decade or two from now when a large cadre of baby boomer–aged physicians retire.

Of course, such a question may be asked of any professional workforce within the United States, given the aging demography of the country. Yet, where medicine is concerned, and because of the wave of reform now sweeping through the healthcare industry, it represents yet another uncertainty injected into a system slowly being turned on its proverbial head. With respect to the topics covered in the remainder of this book, this chapter is an additional reference for considering the issues around other segments of the healthcare workforce. For example, how do changes within the medical profession impact what is happening to other professions such as nursing? In what ways will healthcare organizations have to rethink how they interact and relate to all healthcare workers because of what is happening among physicians? How can and should the "medical model" of care delivery advocated for by a dominant medical profession over the past century, a model focused on waiting until people become sick to deliver care to them, and one acknowledging the supreme authority of the physician in diagnosis and treatment, change because of shifts in physician values, preferences, and experiences? Throughout the remainder of this book, these questions bear closer scrutiny in the context of other workforce developments presented.

In conclusion, although there is uncertainty with the stratification occurring within the US medical profession, there is also reason for optimism about the system impact such stratification brings with it. The future healthcare system in the United States requires ideas and solutions for complex problems from a variety of stakeholders that likely will range from retailers such as Amazon to tech-savvy entrepreneurs such as Google to large, integrated-delivery systems to physicians and other health professionals. Whether or not we have seen the golden age of physician dominance in US healthcare come and go is an open question. But it is clear that physicians will not have the same level of power and control within a reformed US healthcare system to do what they please and in the manner they wish. The implications of an intellectually diverse and nimble profession (i.e., one that can be a source of true innovation for doing things better) in healthcare, even with less power and control, are profound. In this way, an internally stratified medical profession, one that does not necessarily speak or act as one mind, is likely well suited to what the health system will need from it, and in this sense it merits both excitement and further exploration.

References

Abbott, A. (1988). *The system of professions: An essay on the division of expert labor.* Chicago, IL: University of Chicago Press.

Abrams, L. (October 18, 2012). Why we're still waiting on the "yelpification" of health care. *The Atlantic.* Retrieved from http://www.theatlantic.com/health/archive/2012/10/why-were-still-waiting-on-the-yelpification-of-health-care/263815/.

American Medical Association [AMA]. (2013). *Policy research perspectives: new data on physician practice arrangements: private practice remains strong despite shifts toward hospital employment.* Retrieved from http://www.ama-assn.org/ama/pub/advocacy/health-policy/policy-research. page?

Aruguete, M. S., & Roberts, C. A. (2000). *Gender, affiliation, and control in physician-patient encounters, 42*(1-2), 107–118.

Association of American Medical Colleges [AAMC]. (2012). *2012 Physician specialty data book*. Retrieved from https://www.aamc.org/download/313228/data/2012physicianspecialtydata-book.pdf.

Bernstein, A., & Vanderlinde-Kopper, C. (Eds). (2008). *Health care's retail solution*. Retrieved from http://www.boozallen.com/media/file/health-care-retail-solution-sb.pdf.

Bertakis, K. D., Franks, P., & Azari, R. (2003). Effects of physician gender on patient satisfaction. *Journal of the American Medical Women's Association, 58*(2), 69–75.

Bomey, N. (2015). *Anthem to buy Cigna for $54B in mega insurance merger*. Retrieved from http://www.usatoday.com/story/money/2015/07/24/anthem-buy-cigna-mega-insurance-merger/30608995/.

Cochran, A., Hauschild, T., Elder, W. B., Neumayer, L. A., Brasel, K. J., & Crandall M. L. (2013). Perceived gender-based barriers to careers in academic surgery. *American Journal of Surgery, 206*(2), 263–268.

Cohen, S. G., & Bailey, D. E. (1997). What makes teams work: Group effectiveness research from the shop floor to the executive suite. *Journal of Management, 23*(3), 239–290.

Danesh-Meyer, H. V., Deva, N. C., Ku, J. Y., Carol, S. C., Tan, Y. W., & Gamble G. (2007). Differences in practice and personal profiles between male and female ophthalmologists. *Clinical & Experimental Ophthalmology, 35*(4), 318–323.

Deloitte Center for Health Solutions. (2012). *The U.S. health care market: A strategic view of consumer segmentation*. Retrieved from http://www2.deloitte.com/content/dam/Deloitte/us/Documents/life-sciences-health-care/us-lshc-health-care-market-consumer-segmentation.pdf

Dorsey, E. R., Jarjoura, D., & Rutecki, G. W. (2003). Influence of controllable lifestyle on recent trends in specialty choice by US medical students. *Journal of the American Medical Association, 290*(9), 1173–1178.

Drake, B. (March 7, 2014). *Six new findings about millennials*. Pew Research Center. Retrieved from http://www.pewresearch.org/fact-tank/2014/03/07/6-new-findings-about-millennials/.

Freidson, E. (1970). *Profession of medicine: A study of the sociology of applied knowledge*. Chicago, IL: University of Chicago Press.

Glicksman, E. (2013). *Wanting it all: A new generation of doctors places higher value on work-life balance*. Retrieved from https://www.aamc.org/newsroom/reporter/336402/work-life.html.

Herman, B. (February 23, 2013,). 25 highest-paid specialties: Salaries for hospital-employed physicians. *Becker's Healthcare*. Retrieved from http://www.beckershospitalreview.com/compensation-issues/25-highest-paid-physician-specialties-by-hospital-ownership.html.

Hoff, T. J. (1999). The social organization of physicians in a changing HMO. *Work and Occupations, 26*(3), 324–351.

Hoff, T. J. (2004). Doing the same and earning less: Male and female physicians in a new medical specialty. *Inquiry, 41*, 301–315.

Hoff, T. J. (2010). *Practice under pressure: Primary care physicians and their medicine in the twenty-first century*. Piscataway, N.J.: Rutgers University Press.

Hoff, T. J., & Scott, S. (2015). The gendered management realities and talent management imperatives of women physicians. *Health Care Management Review*. Published early online, May 14, doi: 10.1097/HMR.0000000000000069.

Jackson Healthcare. (2013). *Filling the void: 2013 physician outlook & practice trends*. Retrieved from https://www.jacksonhealthcare.com/media/191888/2013physiciantrends-void_ebk0513.pdf.

Jagsi, R., Griffith, K. A., Stewart, A., Sambuco, D., DeCastro, R., & Ubel, P. A. (2012). Gender differences in the salaries of physician researchers. *Journal of the American Medical Association, 307*(22), 2410–2417.

Kass, R. B., Souba, W. W., & Thorndyke, L. E. (2006). Challenges confronting female surgical leaders: Overcoming the barriers. *The Journal of Surgical Research, 132*(2), 179–187.

Katz, B. (2011). Career source: millennial physicians' must-haves: Location, computerized EDs, guaranteed income. *Emergency Medicine News, 33*(1), 30–39.

Larson, M. S. (1977). *The rise of professionalism: A sociological analysis.* Berkeley, CA: University of California Press.

Lo Sasso, A. T., Richards, M. R., Chou, C. F., & Gerber, S. E. (2011). The $16,819 pay gap for newly trained physicians: The unexplained trend of men earning more than women. *Health Affairs (Project Hope), 30*(2), 193–201.

Marley, C. S., Lerner, L. B., Panagopoulos, G., & Kavaler, E. (2011). Personal, professional and financial satisfaction among American women urologists. *International Brazilian Journal of Urology, 37*(2), 187–192; discussion 192–184.

McAlister, C., Jin, Y. P., Braga-Mele, R. DesMarchais, B. F., Buys, Y. M. (2014). Comparison of lifestyle and practice patterns between male and female Canadian ophthalmologists. *Canadian Journal of Ophthalmology, 49*(3), 287–290.

Merton, R. K. (1967). *On theoretical sociology.* New York, NY: The Free Press.

Moore, K. J., Felger, T. A., Larimore, W. L., & Mills, T. (2008). What every physician should know about the RUC. *Family Practice Management, 15*(2), 36–39.

Murgatroyd, L. (1982). Gender and occupational stratification. *The Sociological Review, 30*(4), 574–602.

Ng, E. S., Schweitzer, L., & Lyons, S. T. (2010). New generation, great expectations: A field study of the millennial generation. *Journal of Business and Psychology, 25*(2), 281–292.

The Physicians Foundation. (2010). *Health reform and the decline of physician private practice: A white paper examining the effects of the patient protection and affordable care act on physician practices in the United States.* Retrieved from http://www.physiciansfoundation.org/uploads/default/Health_Reform_and_the_Decline_of_Physician_Private_Practice.pdf.

Reed, D. A., Enders, F., Lindor, R., McClees, M., & Lindor K. D. (2011). Gender differences in academic productivity and leadership appointments of physicians throughout academic careers. *Academic Medicine, 86*(1), 43–47.

Rosenthal, E. (January 18, 2014). Patients' costs skyrocket; specialists' incomes soar. *New York Times.* Retrieved from http://www.nytimes.com/2014/01/19/health/patients-costs-skyrocket-specialists-incomes-soar.html?_r=0.

Roter, D. L., Hall, J. A., & Aoki, Y. (2002). Physician gender effects in medical communication: A meta-analytic review. *Journal of the American Medical Association, 288*(6), 756–764.

Silverman, L. (November 27, 2014). Millennial doctors may be more tech-savvy, but is that better? Retrieved from http://www.npr.org/blogs/health/2014/11/27/366766639/millennial-doctors-may-be-more-tech-savvy-but-is-that-better.

Starr, P. (1982). *The social transformation of American medicine.* New York, NY: Basic Books.

US Bureau of Labor Statistics. (2014a). *Physicians and surgeons*. Retrieved from http://www.bls. gov/ooh/healthcare/physicians-and-surgeons.htm.

US Bureau of Labor Statistics. (2014b). *Women in the labor force: A databook*. Retrieved from http://www.bls.gov/cps/wlf-databook-2013.pdf.

US Department of Labor. (2015). *Employment characteristics of families—2014*. Retrieved from http://www.bls.gov/news.release/famee.toc.htm.

COMMENTARY TO ACCOMPANY CHAPTER 2

Darrell G. Kirch, MD

TIMOTHY HOFF AND HENRY POHL have raised an issue that is both important and timely but has received surprisingly little attention given the remarkable shifts in the physician workforce in recent decades. Major internal and external forces have been reshaping the healthcare industry in ways that have a profound impact on the workforce, affecting everything from physician identity to clinical decision-making, patient care, and interprofessional teams.

As the authors rightly point out, it would be a mistake to think that these changes have been wrought solely by implementation of the Affordable Care Act and an expansion of the government's role in health care. In fact, as described by Victor Fuchs (Fuchs, 2012), multiple forces have been driving health expenditures steadily higher since 1950, including advances in medical technology, the spread of private and public insurance, and a growing and aging population.

As spending grew, the corporatization of healthcare was likely inevitable and in some ways beneficial. In an increasingly complex and high-cost industry, integrating and standardizing care delivery within large organizations has the potential to transform health care to be more consistent, transparent, and effective (Swenson et al., 2010). Similar consolidation has occurred or is underway across major American industries, from airlines to banking to telecommunications. There is no reason to think that healthcare would continue to function like the "last cottage industry" and be immune to this trend. Turning back the clock is simply not an option.

Although transformation may have been inevitable, there is mounting evidence that the rapid pace of change is damaging physician well-being. A recent survey by Tait Shanafelt and colleagues found that 54.5% of US physicians experienced at least one symptom of burnout in 2014—an increase of almost 9% in just 3 years (Shanafelt et al., 2015). The issue of physician burnout is becoming a public health crisis in its own right.

Given the evidence laid out by the authors, the following issues call for further examination and analysis:

- **Physician well-being.** With more than half of our nation's physicians experiencing burnout, we have a problem that cannot be ignored. We know that rapid change accompanied by a personal sense of loss of control contributes to burnout. Maintaining the health of the profession requires a better understanding of both the mechanisms of burnout and the most effective interventions to build physician resilience.
- **Embracing diversity as a driver of excellence.** Although stratification in the physician workforce may lead to varying interests, needs, and day-to-day realities within the profession, the evidence is clear that diverse perspectives also improve collective problem solving and foster innovation (Hong & Page, 2004). As we continue to study how a new generation of physicians is reshaping our workforce, we must embrace diversity as key to improving organizational performance.
- **Emphasizing the role of competencies.** Medical education and physician training have begun to shift away from a focus on accumulating facts toward a greater emphasis on the development and assessment of core professional competencies. As we refine our thinking around competencies and the workforce, we must work to clarify which competencies are core throughout the profession and which are essential for individual specialties and types of practice.
- **New approaches to physician selection and advancement.** Whether admitting a medical student, matching a resident, or hiring a physician, we should employ broader assessment tools to determine the best fit. When the Association of American Medical Colleges (AAMC) revised its MCAT® examination in 2015, it introduced a new section called "Psychological, Social, and Biological Foundations of Behavior" to assess future physicians on their understanding of the social and behavioral determinants of health. We can continue to study other approaches, such as situational judgment tests and structured behavioral interviews, to better assess core competencies at key points in physician development.

Remembering our ethical foundations. Perhaps the greatest question facing the physician workforce today is whether the changes outlined in this chapter will affect our ethical commitments. There is no reason that working in a large organization or pursuing work–life balance should necessarily diminish a physician's dedication to ethical principles, but the danger remains that changes in practice may challenge those commitments. Above all, in the midst of rapid change, physicians must not waver from their core ethical obligations.

References

Fuchs, V. R. (2012). Major trends in the U.S. health economy since 1950. *New England Journal of Medicine 366*(11), 973–977. http://www.nejm.org/doi/full/10.1056/NEJMp1200478.

Hong, L., & Page, S. E. (2004). Groups of diverse problem solvers can outperform groups of high-ability problem solvers. *Proceedings of the National Academy of Sciences of the United States of America 101*(46), 16385–16389. http://doi.org/10.1073/pnas.0403723101.

Shanafelt, T. D., et al. (2015). Changes in burnout and satisfaction with work-life balance in physicians and the general US working population between 2011 and 2014. *Mayo Clinic Proceedings 90*(12), 1600–1613. http://www.mayoclinicproceedings.org/article/S0025-6196%2815%2900716-8/abstract.

Swensen, S. J., et al. (2010). Cottage industry to postindustrial care—the revolution in health care delivery. *New England Journal of Medicine 362*(5), e12. http://www.nejm.org/doi/full/10.1056/NEJMp0911199.

3

TRANSFORMATION OF THE NONPHYSICIAN

HEALTH PROFESSIONS

Joanne Spetz, James F. Cawley, and Jon Schommer

Introduction and Overview

In 2012, the *New York Times* published an editorial titled "When the Doctor is Not Needed." The editorial referred to the widely discussed concern that there has been a long-standing shortage of physicians and that greater health insurance enrollment would exacerbate the problem. But, rather than pointing to expansions of medical schools and residency programs as the only solutions, the editors argued that a broader array of healthcare providers, including nurse practitioners (NPs), physician assistants (PAs), and pharmacists, would provide "a sensible solution to this crisis" (New York Times, 2012).

The *New York Times* editorial board is not alone in seeing opportunities for meeting healthcare needs with nonphysician providers. PricewaterhouseCooper's Health Research Institute identified the use of nonphysicians in patient care as a "top 10" health industry issue of 2015 (PricewaterhouseCooper's Health Research Institute, 2014). They note that consumers appear receptive to seeing NPs and PAs for primary care and minor injuries, as well as to seeing pharmacists for some services. Also, they observe that a growing number of physicians want to work in teams with other providers in order to make more time available for care coordination, time with patients, and work–life balance.

The potential for NPs, PAs, and pharmacists to play an important role in meeting future healthcare needs is defined by their history, education, regulation, and practice. This chapter examines the trajectories of these professions, identifying their distinct but overlapping roles in the healthcare system. Each has experienced some common trends and issues such as increasing educational attainment and the pursuit of greater professional independence. The connections between patterns in the development and maturation of these professions and broader societal and health system trends are highlighted.

Who are Nurse Practitioners, Physician Assistants, and Pharmacists?

Prior to the development of PA and NP education and licensing in the 1960s, the domain of the physician had not been seriously challenged. For more than 100 years, the laws and policies in place with regard to medical practice and authority favored the physician over any other professional licensed to practice medicine. But as the practice of medicine evolves, so do other healthcare professions.

NURSE PRACTITIONERS

NP preparation has its roots in the late 1950s, when registered nurses (RNs) with clinical experience began to collaborate with physicians in the delivery of primary care, particularly in rural areas. The first formal education program for NPs was established in 1965 at the University of Colorado. The curriculum of this program focused on health promotion, disease prevention, and children's health, with an emphasis on care needs in rural areas, and it conferred a certificate of completion. Because NPs could not expect that physicians would be working alongside them in rural communities, they were educated to practice independently. In 2012, there were 154,057 NPs certified to practice in the United States (US Health Resources and Services Administration, 2014); one-half to two-thirds of them worked in primary care (Spetz, Fraher, Li, & Bates, 2015).

Today's NP education programs are graduate-level programs for people who have previously completed a bachelor's degree and are RNs. NP specialties include family practice, pediatrics, women's health, psychiatry, acute care, and community/public health. Nearly all states require new NPs to complete a graduate degree, although most allow previously licensed or certified NPs to continue to practice. In 2012, 86% of NPs reported that their highest education was a master's degree in nursing, 5% held a doctorate in nursing, and 3% held a non-nursing doctorate (US Health Resources and Services Administration, 2014). There are several national certifying organizations for NPs; most states require national certification to obtain an initial NP license. NP education programs have grown over the past decade, with approximately 15,000 people completing NP education programs in the 2012-2013 academic year (American Association of Nurse Practitioners [AANP], 2015a), which is more than double the 6,611 graduates in 2003 (US Health Resources and Services Administration, 2013a).

The NP workforce is less diverse than many other health occupations, with 86% being non-Hispanic white and 93% being female (US Health Resources and Services Administration, 2014). The average age of the NP workforce in 2014 was 48 years (US Health Resources and Services Administration, 2014).

PHYSICIAN ASSISTANTS

The PA was a workforce idea created by physicians in 1965 as a policy response to a shortage and uneven distribution of generalist physicians (Cawley, Cawthon, & Hooker, 2012). The PA profession was based on the legal premise that PAs would have a defined relationship with physicians and would practice medicine in connection with their physician colleagues. The close practice connection of PAs with physicians has led to widespread acceptance and utilization of PAs in a broad range of clinical practice settings and specialties. There are approximately 100,000 PAs in the present workforce (US Health Resources and Services Administration, 2013b), and about 25% of PAs practice in the primary care specialties of family medicine, general internal medicine, and general pediatrics.

When the PA profession began, education was through a variety of certificate and degree programs. Now, education is at the master's degree level, with 196 existing accredited educational programs and 77 more in development (Accreditation Review Commission on Education for the Physician Assistant, 2015). Although all PAs are trained in the generalist model, PAs are employed in primary care, specialty, and subspecialty medicine (American Academy of Physician Assistants [AAPA], 2014). PA curricula are largely modeled after medical education, with 1 year devoted to basic and clinical sciences and 1 year of clinical practicum rotations. To qualify for licensure in all states, PA graduates must pass the Physician Assistant National Certifying Examination. The 2014 graduating cohort was 7,200 (estimated); this number is projected to increase to 9,000 annual graduates by 2020 (Hooker, Cawley, & Leinweber, 2010; Hooker, Cawley, & Everett, 2011).

There has been a gender shift in the PA workforce since the mid-1990s. In 2015, approximately 66% of working PAs were women, which is a marked contrast to the 1970s when most were male and ex-military medical corpsmen. In 2011, about two thirds of matriculates to PA education were female and the median age at graduation

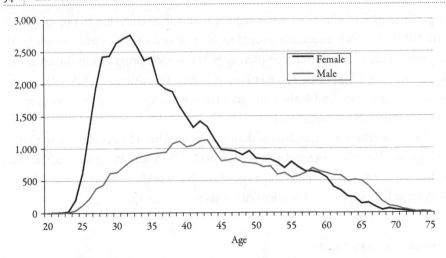

FIGURE 3.1 Number of Physician Assistants, by Age and Sex, 2013.

Note: Source data from Hooker, R. S., & Muchow, A. (2014). The 2013 census of licensed physician assistants. *Journal of the American Association of Physician Assistants, 27,* 1–6.

was 29 years (Hooker et al., 2010; Hooker et al., 2011). This demographic shift may account for the falling proportion of PAs working in rural and medically underserved practice settings (13% in 2015). About 80% of all PAs are younger than age 55, making this one of the more youthful health professions (see Figure 3.1). The median age of PAs in clinical practice is 38 years. PA programs continue to attract large numbers of well-qualified applicants; the ratio of applicant to accepted student was 3.4:1 in 2014.

PHARMACISTS

Pharmacists serve important roles to help ensure that the use of medicines results in the highest likelihood of achieving desired health and economic outcomes. In addition to the safe and efficient distribution and provision of medications, pharmacists offer clinical expertise regarding selection, handling, preparation, procurement, and utilization of medications (Higby, 1996) and, more recently, ensuring that drugs reach their full potential for patients in society (Schondelmeyer, 2009). There were 250,652 individuals licensed as pharmacists in the United States in 2014 (Gaither, Schommer, Doucette, Kreling, & Mott, 2015).

Pharmacists are trained with a focus in medication therapy management, including the management of risks as medications are utilized by patients. Pharmacists are educated to conduct patient assessments, identify drug-related problems, develop care plans, and provide follow-up evaluations (Maine, Knapp, & Scheckelhoff, 2013). Increased utilization of pharmacists in various practice settings has been identified as a way to improve access to care for patients and to enhance care coordination

(Knapp, Paavola, Maine, Sorofman, & Politzer, 1998). Pharmacists are widely distributed throughout the United States, including where there are shortages of health professionals and in rural areas. Most pharmacists work in settings that have extended hours of operation every day of the week (McGinnis, Strand, & Webb, 2010). For many Americans, the pharmacy is their most accessible option for healthcare, with approximately 90% of the population living within 5 miles of one of the 67,000 pharmacies in the United States.

Figure 3.2 presents the total number of pharmacy graduates for the years 1965 to 2013. As with many other health degrees, the number of pharmacy degrees conferred in the 1970s increased in response to federal capitation payments designed to stimulate growth in clinical education. This capitation was discontinued in the early 1980s, and the number of pharmacy degrees conferred dropped but then recovered to a straight-line growth pattern. Between 1995 and 2004, many schools of pharmacy went through a conversion to the Doctor of Pharmacy (PharmD) degree, which is discussed in more detail later in this chapter. During that time, class sizes were decreased and, in some years, no graduates were produced at some schools as the conversion took place.

From 2007 to the present, there has been an expansion of pharmacy schools and increases in the number of pharmacy degrees conferred per year. Part of this expansion is in response to opportunities created by healthcare reform and some may be due to the adoption of a professional doctoral program at universities as a way to

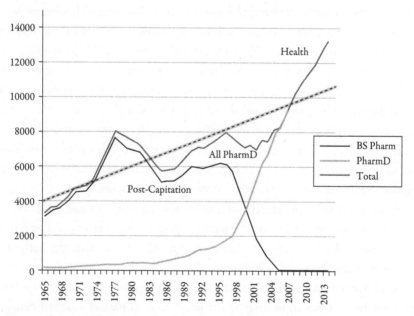

FIGURE 3.2 Pharmacy Degrees Conferred, by Type of Degree, 1966–2013.
Note: Source data from American Association of Colleges of Pharmacy. (2014). *Fall 2013 profile of pharmacy students*. Alexandria, Virginia: American Association of Colleges of Pharmacy.

build prestige and meet perceived public need. Currently, there is debate in the profession about whether the expansion of programs might lead to future oversupply (Brown, 2013; Knapp & Schommer, 2013; Romanelli & Tracy, 2015).

The pharmacy profession has changed from a male-majority profession to a female-majority profession. Since 1985, the number of female graduates has outnumbered male graduates. In 2000, 43% of all licensed pharmacists in the United States were female. In 2014, 53% were female (Gaither et al., 2015). Males and females do not differ regarding the proportions in management positions (29% and 28%, respectively). Recent research has concluded that the position of pharmacist is among the most egalitarian of all US professions (Goldin & Katz, in press), with a low gender earnings gap and a only modest wage penalty for part-time work.

Power, Work, and Control in These Three Professions

PROFESSIONAL CONTROL AND INDEPENDENCE

Most health professions are regulated by state licensing boards; NPs, PAs, and pharmacists must be certified or licensed by the state in which they practice in order to work in their profession. More than three fourths of health workers are employed in licensed occupations. These occupations also are often subject to regulations regarding their scope of practice: whether they must be supervised or collaborate with other professionals and whether they can be reimbursed directly by insurance companies (Kleiner & Park, 2010). When there is overlap in the potential roles of health professionals, or if licensure is tied to that of other health professionals, occupational licensure and regulation is more controversial, and greater variation can be found across states (Kleiner, Marier, Park, & Wing, 2014). The roles of NPs, PAs, and physicians overlap substantially, particularly in primary care and office-based specialty care, whereas pharmacists' roles have historically been viewed as complementary to the other professions. Thus, it is not surprising that NPs and PAs face greater variation in regulatory requirements for licensure/certification to practice across states than pharmacists.

State regulations for pharmacists designate how pharmacists and prescribers can enter into voluntary collaborative pharmacy practice agreements and assign ultimate authority on the scope of pharmacist-provided services to the authorizing prescribers. These laws and regulations allow pharmacists to provide patient care services and activities for groups of patients, including prescribing drugs or ordering laboratory tests, if put in writing by the prescribers as part of a signed collaborative pharmacy practice agreement. In addition, a few states, including California and North Carolina, have established provisions for pharmacists to independently engage in prescribing some medications and ordering tests to monitor medication effectiveness and side effects.

PAs share an interdependent relationship with physicians, sociologically described as "negotiated performance autonomy" (Schneller, 1978). Most jurisdictions license and regulate PAs through state medical boards, but 11 states have regulatory bodies strictly for PAs. PA scope of practice corresponds to the supervising physician's practice and specialty, and it varies according to their training, experience, facility policy, practice needs, and state law. PAs have prescribing authority in all states, although laws vary with regard to certain prescribing privileges and supervisory requirements. In some rural areas where physicians are in short supply, PAs work semiautonomously, conferring with their supervising physicians as needed and as required by law (Henry, Hooker, & Yates, 2011l Davis, Radix, Cawley, & Hooker, 2015).

NPs, in contrast, view themselves as independent healthcare providers; the initial conception of the profession required independence because it focused on rural care where physicians might not be present. NPs believe that as nurses they are empowered to act independently, with the authority to practice and prescribe medications without physician oversight. NPs want their reimbursement rates to be brought up to physician rates for a "like service" (Safriet, 1992). In 2015, 22 states allowed NPs to practice and prescribe medications without physician collaboration or supervision (AANP, 2015b). The remaining states restricted NP practice in a myriad of ways; for example, some do not allow NPs to prescribe any medications, some prohibit prescribing scheduled drugs, some require physician supervision, and some demand that a physician review a fixed share of patient charts. NPs have been actively advocating for the removal of collaboration and supervision requirements, and at times they have been overtly hostile toward professional physician associations (and vice-versa).

There has been a trend since 2000 toward regulatory reforms that allow NPs and PAs greater practice independence (Gadbois, Miller, Tyler, & Intrator, 2014). This trend is expected to accelerate, due to increasing recognition of the potential for NPs and PAs to play a greater role in meeting healthcare needs (National Association of Community Health Centers, 2013; Doescher, Andrilla, Skillman, Morgan, & Kaplan, 2014;) and the influential Institute of Medicine report on the role of nursing in meeting healthcare needs, which recommended that regulations allow nurses to practice to the fullest extent of their education (Institute of Medicine, 2011).

EDUCATION UPSKILLING

Increasing complexity in the clinical components and contextual environment of healthcare delivery has spurred some professions, including pharmacists, NPs, certified registered nurse anesthetists, and physical therapists, to move toward higher educational standards. For example, to help ensure pharmacists' capacity for their emerging roles in healthcare, the pharmacy profession has increased its focus on direct patient care and collaborative practice, resulting in reforms for both pharmacist training and practice (Schommer, Cline, & Larson, 2005; Knapp & Knapp, 2009; Council on Credentialing in Pharmacy, 2010; Schommer et al., 2010; Maine et al., 2013). In 2004, the Accreditation Council for Pharmacy Education standards for five-year bachelor's of pharmacy programs expired and the Doctor of Pharmacy (PharmD) became the sole accredited professional degree for pharmacy in the United States. This change was motivated by recognition that pharmacy education needed to change to fulfill new roles in healthcare and to improve preparedness for patient-focused care. PharmD programs had existed for decades but grew markedly in the early 1990s after the change in accreditation requirements was announced (Figure 3.2).

In 2014, 50% of pharmacists working in medication dispensing and patient care positions held a PharmD degree (Gaither et al., 2015). Growing numbers of pharmacists also complete specialized residency training, and integrated healthcare organizations often require residency training for hiring (Gather et al., 2015). It is estimated that 4,700 (34%) of the roughly 14,000 pharmacy school graduates in 2014 sought residency training after graduation (ASHP Residency Resource Center, www.ashp.org). The overall goal of the education upskilling for pharmacists was to increase the profession's capacity for medication management and patient-centered, personalized care. A substantial body of evidence has demonstrated that when pharmacists provide care to patients with a variety of chronic conditions, patient care improves and costs decrease (Isasi & Krofah, 2015; Schommer, Planas, & Doucette, 2015). Because of their skills and training, pharmacists are ideally positioned to provide an access point for community-focused primary care services in areas where this is limited access to other primary care providers.

This trend among pharmacists may be specific to that profession in terms of the motivation to move to the doctoral degree. In other professions, the reasons for a transition to the doctorate are less obvious. For NPs, physical therapists, and perhaps for PAs, a shift to the doctoral degree may not change their scope of clinical practice. Thus, this trend raises the question of the motivation for doctoral degrees among some of the health professions and suggests that the root of such trends may lie within higher education programs rather than within the professions themselves.

In 2004, the American Association of Colleges of Nursing (AACN) approved a position statement that supported adoption of the doctor of nursing practice (DNP) degree as the entry-level standard for all advanced practice RNs, including NPs, by 2020 (Martsolf, Auerbach, Spetz, Pearson, & Muchow, 2015). However, the AACN statement has not been followed by changes in accreditation or licensing requirements, with the exception of nurse anesthesia, for which educational programs must offer a DNP by 2025. In 2013, only 25% of advanced practice RN programs offered the option for baccalaureate-educated RNs to go directly to a DNP. More than half of such programs offered a masters-to-doctorate program.

Those who support more advanced education for healthcare providers, including NPs and pharmacists, note that there is a greater need for skills in patient care management, development and execution of quality improvement programs, and stronger engagement in organizational policy. Those who have opposed doctoral requirements—primarily for NPs—have argued that there is no evidence that doctoral education leads to better patient care and that doctoral education is more expensive (Martsolf et al., 2015). Some critics have argued that the proliferation of doctorate degrees—and the title "Doctor"—will lead to confusion among patients and is an overt challenge to the primacy of physicians (Harris, 2011). In light of this ongoing discussion, it is likely that the education of NPs will remain in flux as long as uncertainty about the value of the DNP remains. For PAs, entry-level doctoral programs are on the horizon. The anticipated introduction of one such program at Baylor College of Medicine, which is a prominent academic health center, will likely lead to additional entry-level doctoral programs. Because the practice scope of PAs is not typically a function of formal education, a key question is whether doctoral training will have any effect on the roles and clinical capabilities of PAs in practice.

Current and Potential Roles in Healthcare

INTEGRATED AND TEAM CARE

Interest in NPs, PAs, and pharmacists has risen due to increased attention to integrated care practices that can improve patient care without increasing costs, as well as growing efforts to expand access to care through the use of nonphysician providers. The patient-centered medical home brings together professionals from multiple specialties to work as a team to meet patient needs (Willard & Bodenheimer, 2012). These teams often include physicians, PAs, NPs, medical assistants, RNs, and pharmacists. Not only can team-based care improve quality; it also can mitigate current and projected shortages of primary care physicians (Auerbach et al., 2013; Bodenheimer & Smith, 2013; Green, Savin, & Lu, 2013). Within the Department of Veterans Affairs, Department of Defense, and Indian Health Service, pharmacists manage patient care when medications are the primary treatment. This includes starting, stopping, and adjusting medications; ordering and interpreting laboratory tests; and coordinating follow-up care. NPs are the primary care providers in hundreds of retail clinics nationwide, where they treat common conditions such as ear infections, urinary tract infections, and bronchitis at a lower cost than other settings. The education of PAs makes them well-suited to providing care in a range of primary and specialty areas (New York Times, 2012).

A substantial body of research demonstrates that PAs and NPs provide patient care of similar quality as physicians within specific types of care and scopes of practice (Office of Technology Assessment, 1986; Newhouse et al., 2011). PAs in primary care report less time consulting with physicians as they gain more experience working in that physician's practice (Cawley & Bush, 2015). Numerous studies have demonstrated comparable performance between NPs and primary care physicians on clinical outcomes, including reduction of symptoms, improvement in health and functional status, and mortality (Horrocks, Anderson, & Salisbury, 2002; Naylor & Kurtzman, 2010). Also, some studies have shown higher satisfaction among patients seen by NPs (Hooker, Cipher, & Sekscenski, 2005; Jennings, Clifford, Fox, O'Connell, & Gardner, 2014).

NPs and PAs are neither perfect substitutes for each other nor perfect substitutes for physicians. Each of these professions has different educational experiences and different views of their role in providing healthcare. NP education is within a specific area of practice, such as adult primary care, pediatrics, mental health, family care, or acute care. Most NPs are prepared in one of the primary care areas, and at least half work in primary care (Spetz et al., 2015). In contrast, PAs are prepared as medical generalists, and thus they are able to adapt to the clinical practice setting of the physician. In the course of a career, at least half of PAs have changed specialties more than once over a theoretical 35-year professional career (Hooker et al., 2010). This role flexibility is believed to contribute to a high degree of job satisfaction and the retention of PAs in clinical practice (Marvelle & Kraditor, 1999; LaBarbera, 2004; Hooker et al., 2010).

Although the role of the pharmacist is comparatively distinct from those of physicians and other providers, pharmacists are being integrated into systems of care that utilize their expertise beyond traditional roles. New roles for pharmacists include the following:

- Serving in expanded roles such as medication care coordination within primary care teams (American Society of Health-System Pharmacists, 1999; Dettloff, Glosner, & Moroney, 2009; Dobson et al., 2009; Webb, 2009; Gebhart, 2010; Manolakis & Skelton, 2010)
- Working within chronic disease management teams (Goff & Greenland, 2009; Lipton, 2009; Manolakis & Skelton, 2010)
- Being responsible for ensuring optimal medication therapy outcomes through medication therapy management service provision (Lewin, 2005; Smith & Clancy, 2006; Hassol & Shoemaker, 2008; Joint Commission of

Pharmacy Practitioners, 2008; Barnett et al., 2009; Manolakis & Skelton, 2010; Owen & Burns, 2010; Isetts, Brummel, de Oliveira, & Moen, 2012; Wittayanukorn et al., 2013; Santschi et al., 2014; Isasi & Krofah, 2015)

Increased efficiencies in pharmacists' medication-providing roles have been achieved through the use of advanced logistics (e.g., centralized fill), technicians, and technology (e.g., bar code scanning, e-prescribing, robotics) (US Health Resources and Services Administration, 2008). This has made it possible for pharmacists to take on additional responsibilities and contribute more generally to the care team. In fact, a recent report suggested that pharmacists' roles are evolving to include providing direct patient care as members of integrated healthcare provider teams and that this has the potential to improve health outcomes (Isasi & Krofah, 2015). The report concluded that "the integration of pharmacists into team-based models of care could potentially lead to improved health outcomes. To realize that prospect, states should consider engaging in coordinated efforts to address the greatest challenges pharmacists face: restrictions in [collaborative practice agreements], recognition of pharmacists as health care providers to ensure compensation for direct patient care services, and access to health [information technology] systems" (Isasi & Krofah, 2015).

RETAIL CLINICS AND OTHER NONTRADITIONAL SETTINGS

Community pharmacies are becoming increasingly important sites of care, both in the fulfillment of prescriptions and in the growth of retail-based clinics. Pharmacists are the most frequently encountered health professionals for many patients. These pharmacists have become public health advocates in areas such as health screening, health improvement programs, and immunization services. It is estimated that 87% of US pharmacists are trained to administer vaccines, and 52 states and territories permit them to do so (American Pharmacists Association, 2015). Community pharmacy settings afford the opportunity to coordinate self-care behaviors that are in addition to, or complement, prescribed therapies, including over-the-counter drugs and nutritional supplements. For patients who are under the care of multiple prescribers and who utilize multiple healthcare settings, community pharmacies are ideal for improving continuity and coordination of chronic care because many patients visit community pharmacies at frequent and regular intervals.

Within pharmacies, there is a growing number of retail clinics, which offer diagnosis and treatment for common, low-acuity conditions. In 2011, there were more than 1,800 clinics (Japsen, 2015), in which NPs are the primary providers of healthcare services (Deloitte Center for Health Solutions, 2009). There is substantial evidence that retail clinics provide the type of care in which they specialize (generally low-acuity services such as diagnosis of basic upper respiratory tract infection) efficiently, reduce the cost of healthcare, and achieve high levels of patient satisfaction (Thygeson, Van Vorst, Maciosek, & Solberg, 2008; Hunter, Weber, Morreale, & Wall, 2009; Mehrotra et al., 2009; Weinick, Burns, & Mehrotra, 2010). However, state laws that restrict the scope of practice of NPs—specifically the requirement that NPs collaborate with or be supervised by physicians—have been shown to reduce the cost savings achieved by retail clinics (Spetz, Parente, Town, & Bazarko, 2013).

HOSPITAL AND HOSPITALIST ROLES

Pharmacists, NPs, and PAs are engaged in broader roles in hospitals than in the past. Incentives to reduce rehospitalizations have brought attention to the need to manage medications more effectively between the hospital and the postdischarge setting. Care of a patient who is being discharged from a hospital would be enhanced by sharing of information between the hospital pharmacist and community pharmacist. Pharmacist-to-pharmacist referral involving communication between different pharmacy and healthcare settings is a necessary step for enhancing access to pharmacist-provided patient care (Brummel et al., 2014). The typical patient still encounters gaps in care and endures duplication of effort by pharmacists who do not have complete information at the time they provide patient care services.

NPs and PAs also work in hospitals, playing a variety of roles. PAs often provide care within hospital operating rooms, emergency departments, critical care units, and inpatient and outpatient units of hospitals (AAPA, 2014). They can serve as assistants during surgery, work with substantial autonomy in emergency departments, and provide other acute and ancillary services. NPs can specialize in acute care when they receive their education and often work side-by-side with hospitalist physicians. NPs and PAs also can play greater roles in facilitating effective transitions between the hospital and postdischarge settings, by providing predischarge education, care coordination, and home visitation. Multiple models of care using PAs and NPs have been proven to reduce rehospitalizations (Kocher & Adashi, 2011), including the transitional care model (Naylor et al., 1999; Naylor et al., 2004) and the care transitions program (Coleman et al., 2004).

Implications for Practice

Ongoing primary care shortages, increasing demand for care due to population growth and aging and the implementation of the Patient Protection and Affordable

Care Act, the imperative to improve quality of care, and demand to increase the value of care are converging to bring the roles of PAs, pharmacists, and NPs forward across numerous settings. To optimize the employment of these professions in the enhancement and expansion of care, changes in (a) education, (b) scope of practice regulations, and (c) payment policies may be required.

EDUCATION CHANGES

Pharmacist, NP, and PA education will need greater depth in care coordination and care management, interprofessional teamwork, and evidence-based practice in order to meet the demands of the rapidly changing healthcare system. Many education programs for these professions do not include content in these areas. For example, pharmacist education at this time does not focus on diagnosis and initial prescribing of treatments, although a growing number of states are considering permitting pharmacists to prescribe contraceptives and other medications, as well as to manage medications more directly.

The DNP degree for NPs is intended to address the need for greater knowledge of the healthcare system's organization and financing, critical assessment of research, development and implementation of evidence-based practices, and other competencies that will be increasingly needed. Diffusion of these programs has been rapid, but a small share of NPs has completed such education thus far. A comparable education pathway for PAs includes the more than 70 PA postgraduate residency programs, most of which are hospital-based and do not confer a degree. Doctoral degrees for entry-level PA education may be in development soon.

SCOPE OF PRACTICE REGULATIONS

States have the authority to establish their own regulations regarding licensing and scope of practice of health professions. A number of analyses suggest that allowing NPs, PAs, and pharmacists to practice with greater autonomy might increase access to care and reduce the cost of healthcare (Hooker & Muchow, 2015). Practice autonomy in primary care has been authorized for PAs who practice in closed healthcare systems such as the Veterans Administration (Petzel, 2013), and NPs can practice without physician supervision or collaboration in nearly half of US states (AANP, 2015b).

The impact of NP scope of practice regulations has been studied more than those of other professions. Restrictive scope of practice regulations for NPs have been linked to lower utilization of primary care services (Stange, 2014) and higher costs in retail healthcare clinics (Spetz et al., 2013). It is likely that restrictions on the practice of PAs have similar effects on access and costs. Greater autonomy would support a greater degree of utilization of PAs and NPs in primary care to fill gaps in the supply of primary care physicians. Although there is no indication that PAs are seeking a more independent practice stance, there is evidence that PAs, particularly those in primary care, enjoy high levels of practice autonomy and typically have their own patient panels. Career pathways for PAs appear to be broadening, especially for those employed in large health systems where management roles such as managing large PA and NP departments appear to be emerging. Pharmacy practice acts also will need to be updated in light of pharmacists' new roles and to reduce state-to-state variation in regulations (Isasi & Krofah, 2015).

Healthcare organizations also control the practice of PAs, NPs, and pharmacists, by establishing their own rules about what each provider can and cannot do. These rules and restrictions undermine professional authority, which is based on the idea that professional peers are best suited to judge performance and determine scope of practice (Sitkin & Sutcliffe, 1991). However, if legal liability rests with the organization, either in place of or in addition to the provider, organizations may seek to control risk through bureaucratic restrictions. Some hospitals do not permit NPs and PAs to oversee patient care, for example. Organizations might restrict the ability of pharmacists to manage medications, even when state regulations permit them to do so. Variation in the roles of health professionals across healthcare organizations creates confusion for providers and patients alike.

PAYMENT POLICIES

Payment regulations for NPs, PAs, and pharmacists vary across states, as well as across federal health payment programs. Medicare pays NPs and PAs at 85% of the physician fee schedule, and Medicaid payment rates differ from state to state (AAPA, 2013; Chapman, Wides, & Spetz, 2010). Within Medicare, PAs and NPs can bill their services as being provided "incident to" physician services at 100% of the physician reimbursement rate. Nearly all private insurers reimburse services provided by PAs and NPs, but some require that services be billed under the name of the physician. Other insurers allow NPs and PAs to bill independently.

Greater use of pharmacists, NPs, and PAs in healthcare teams may be hindered by payment regulations that focus on fee-for-service reimbursement. In fee-for-service reimbursement, providers must attend to the payment that will be received for each service, as compared with the time dedicated to providing the service. New payment approaches, such as bundled payments and value-based payments, place greater emphasis on the outcomes achieved by services rather than the number of services. These approaches also may facilitate team-based care by decoupling the reimbursement from the specific provider of care. These new payment mechanisms will be particularly important for providers who do not often bill independently for services, such as pharmacists. As pharmacists become more engaged in medication management and coordination, payment structures will be required to ensure that this expanded role is appropriately reimbursed (Isasi & Krofah, 2015).

Implications for Theory and Research

Although there are overlapping competencies among physicians, NPs, PAs, and pharmacists, each of these professions has distinct knowledge and skills, and thus can play a distinct role. Although major research reports and policy analyses often consider PAs and NPs to be equivalent in ambulatory practice roles (Office of Technology Assessment, 1986), and PAs and NPs have similar views about their roles (Hooker & Freeborn, 1995), there are important differences. Pharmacists have a more clearly distinct role, but as they become more engaged in patient care and medication management, overlap with physician responsibilities will increase.

The evolution of new roles of pharmacists, PAs, and NPs will need to be evaluated to determine the optimal placement of each of these professions. The theoretical and practice foundations of each profession need explication so that each group understands the approach of the other. In addition, the economic impact of utilization of these professionals both in independent roles and within teams requires evaluation. Thus far, for example, there has been little exploration of the differences in preventive content of primary care service delivery by NPs, PAs, and family physicians. Early findings show that NPs and PAs engage in health education interventions to a greater degree than do physicians (Ritsema, Bingenheimer, Scholting, & Cawley, 2014). Although many advocates argue that expanded use of NPs, PAs, and pharmacists will inevitably improve quality of care and lower costs, there is a need for research that rigorously tests whether there is a causal relationship between such expanded use and desired outcomes.

The relationship between professional education and the capacity of pharmacists, NPs, and PAs to effectively fulfill their new responsibilities is not clearly delineated. While new educational programs such as the DNP degree for NPs and the entry-level doctorate for PAs are expanding, the value of these programs has not yet been demonstrated in research. Thus far, there is no evidence that individuals educated in such programs have demonstrably different clinical roles than those trained at the master's level. In addition, the effectiveness of new educational modalities for providing additional knowledge to pharmacists, NPs, and PAs has not been evaluated adequately. Finally, there is an inadequate body of knowledge regarding the roles of NPs and PAs in clinical settings where there has been increasing demand and utilization, for example in inpatient house staff settings, critical care units, certain subspecialties, and urgent care settings.

In order to further establish pathways for access to patient care provided by PAs, NPs, and pharmacists, we propose that the application of collaboration theory might be useful for closing gaps that currently exist between organizations in the healthcare system (Schommer, Planas, & Doucette, 2015). Collaboration theory provides guidance about how joint decision-making among autonomous key stakeholders can be used to resolve planning problems and/or manage issues related to planning and development across organizations. Working together enables the participating organizations to create and capture mutual advantages that translate into positive outcomes and more efficient management. Such an approach will be associated with risk and will require trust between participating organizations. In addition, such progress is likely to require updating and contemporizing practice acts and other statutes to allow these practitioners to practice at maximum capacity within new models of care. Furthermore, payment and documentation systems, incentives, and contracting approaches will need to change to develop proper reimbursement and accounting for these new roles. Leadership is needed at multiple levels, including national, state, professional, academic, and organizational, for creating (a) collaborative performance systems, (b) information sharing, (c) decision synchronization, (d) incentive alignment, and (e) integrated processes.

Conclusions

Nonphysician health professions, including NPs, pharmacists, and PAs, have played an important role in healthcare delivery for decades, and their importance to the US healthcare system is increasing. Each profession has a unique history, but all have some overlapping competencies and roles with physicians and with each other. The growing need for more efficient patient-centered healthcare will likely lead to more visible roles for nonphysician professions, both as independent providers and as members of teams.

In order to optimally leverage the unique knowledge and skills each of these professions offers, policymakers need to revisit licensing, scope of practice, and payment regulations. Organizations that employ PAs, NPs, and pharmacists also need to examine their internal policies to ensure they do not establish unneeded barriers to patient care. We propose that the contributions of NPs, PAs, and pharmacists can be enhanced by creating and implementing (a) collaborative work systems, (b) information sharing, (c) decision synchronization, (d) incentive alignment, and (e) integrated payment processes within healthcare systems. As the healthcare system continues its evolution, and these professions grow into new roles, evaluation and research will identify the impact of these professions in a transformed healthcare environment and the pathway for the future of each.

References

Accreditation Review Commission on Education for the Physician Assistant. (2015). *Program Data* (April 2015). Retrieved from http://www.arc-pa.com/acc_programs/program_data.html

American Academy of Physician Assistants (AAPA). (2013). *Reimbursement issues: Third-party reimbursement for PAs.* Alexandria, Virginia: American Academy of Physician Assistants.

AAPA. (2014). *AAPA Survey of Physician Assistants, 2013.* Alexandria, Virginia: American Academy of Physician Assistants.

American Association of Nurse Practitioners (AANP). (2015a). *NP facts.* Retrieved from http://www.aanp.org/images/documents/about-nps/npfacts.pdf

AANP. (2015b). *State nurse practice acts and administrative rules.* Retrieved from http://www.aanp.org/images/documents/state-leg-reg/stateregulatorymap.pdf

American Pharmacists Association. (2015). *Immunization center.* Retrieved from http://www.pharmacist.com/immunization-center

American Society of Health-System Pharmacists. (1999). ASHP statement on the pharmacist's role in primary care. *American Journal of Health Systems Pharmacy, 56*(16), 1665–1667.

Auerbach, D. I., Chen, P. G., Friedberg, M. W., Reid, R., Lau, C., Buerhaus, P. I., & Mehrotra, A. (2013). Nurse-managed health centers and patient-centered medical homes could mitigate expected primary care physician shortage. *Health Affairs, 32*(11), 1933–1941.

Barnett, M. J., Frank, J., Wehring, H., Newland, B., VonMuenster, S., Kumbera, P., Perry, P. J. (2009). Analysis of pharmacist-provided medication therapy management (MTM) services in community pharmacies over 7 years. *Journal of Managed Care Pharmacy, 15*(1), 18–31.

Bodenheimer, T. S., & Smith, M. D. (2013). Primary care: proposed solutions to the physician shortage without training more physicians. *Health Affairs, 32*(11), 1881–1886.

Brown, D. L. (2013). A looming joblessness crisis for new pharmacy graduates and the implications it holds for the academy. *American Journal of Pharmacy Education, 77*(5), 90.

Brummel, A., Lustig, A., Westrich, K., Evans, M. A., Plank, G. S., Penso, J., & Dubois, R. W. (2014). Best practices: Improving patient outcomes and costs in an ACO through comprehensive medication therapy management. *Journal of Managed Care and Specialty Pharmacy, 20*(12), 1152–1158.

Cawley, J. F., & Bush, E. (2015). Levels of supervision among practicing physician assistants. *Journal of the American Association of Physician Assistants, 28*(1), 61–62.

Cawley, J. F., Cawthon, E., & Hooker, R. S. (2012). Origins of the physician assistant movement in the United States. *Journal of the American Academy of Physician Assistants, 25*(12), 36–40.

Chapman, S. A., Wides, C. D., & Spetz, J. (2010). Payment regulations for advanced practice nurses: Implications for primary care. *Policy, Politics, & Nursing Practice, 11*(2), 89–98.

Coleman, E. A., Smith, J. D., Frank, J. C., Min, S. J., Parry, C., & Kramer, A. M. (2004). Preparing patients and caregivers to participate in care delivered across settings: The Care Transitions Intervention. *Journal of the American Geriatrics Society, 52*(11), 1817–1825.

Council on Credentialing in Pharmacy. (2010). Scope of contemporary pharmacy practice: Roles, responsibilities, and functions of pharmacists and pharmacy technicians. *Journal of the American Pharmacist Association, 50*(2), e35–e69.

Davis, A., Radix, S. M., Cawley, J. F., & Hooker, R. S. (2015). Access and innovation in a time of rapid change: Physician assistant scope of practice. *Annals of Health Law, 23,* 286–336.

Deloitte Center for Health Solutions. (2009). *Retail clinics: Update and implications*: Deloitte Development LLC.

Dettloff, R. W., Glosner, P., & Moroney, S. M. (2009). Establishing the role of the pharmacist in the patient-centered medical home. The opportunity is now. *Journal of Pharmacy Technology, 25*(5), 287–291.

Dobson, R. T., Taylor, J. G., Henry, C. J., Lachaine, J., Zello, G. A., Keegan, D. L., & Forbes, D. A. (2009). Taking the lead: Community pharmacists' perception of their role potential within the primary care team. *Research in Social and Administrative Pharmacy, 5*(4), 327–336.

Doescher, M. P., Andrilla, C. H. A., Skillman, S. M., Morgan, P., & Kaplan, L. (2014). The contribution of physicians, physician assistants, and nurse practitioners toward rural primary care: Findings from a 13-state survey. *Medical Care, 52*(6), 549–556.

Gadbois, E. A., Miller, E. A., Tyler, D., & Intrator, O. (2014). Trends in state regulation of nurse practitioners and physician assistants, 2001 to 2010. *Medical Care Research and Review, 72*(2), 200–219.

Gaither, C. A., Schommer, J. C., Doucette, W. R., Kreling, D. H., & Mott, D. A. (January 31, 2015). *Final report of the 2014 National Pharmacist Workforce Survey*. Paper presented at the Pharmacy Workforce Center, Alexandria, VA.

Gebhart, F. (2010). Put pharmacists on primary care team, says Perdue CMO. *Drug Topics, 154*(1), 23.

Goff, D. C., & Greenland, P. (2009). The change we need in health care. *Archives of Internal Medicine, 169*(8), 737–739.

Goldin, C., & Katz, L. F. (in press). A most egalitarian profession: Pharmacy and the evolution of a family-friendly occupation. *Journal of Labor Economics.*

Green, L. V., Savin, S., & Lu, Y. (2013). Primary care physician shortages could be eliminated through use of teams, nonphysicians, and electronic communication. *Health Affairs, 32*(1), 11–19.

Harris, G. (October 1, 2011). When the nurse wants to be called doctor. *The New York Times.* Retrieved from http://www.nytimes.com/2011/10/02/health/policy/02docs.html?_r=0

Hassol, A., & Shoemaker, S. J. (2008). *Exploratory Research on Medication Therapy Management: Final Report.* Cambridge, MA: Abt Associates. Retrieved from https://www.cms.gov/Research-Statistics-Data-and-Systems/Statistics-Trends-and-Reports/Reports/downloads/blackwell.pdf

Henry, L. R., Hooker, R. S., & Yates, K. L. (2011). The role of physician assistants in rural health care: A systematic review of the literature. *The Journal of Rural Health, 27*(2), 220–229.

Higby, G. J. (1996). From compounding to caring: An abridged history of American pharmacy. *Pharmaceutical Care,* 18–45. New York, NY: Chapman & Hall.

Hooker, R. S., Cawley, J. F., & Everett, C. M. (2011). Predictive modeling the physician assistant supply: 2010-2025. *Public Health Reports, 126*(5), 708–716.

Hooker, R. S., Cawley, J. F., & Leinweber, W. (2010). Career flexibility of physician assistants and the potential for more primary care. *Health Affairs, 29*(5), 880–886.

Hooker, R. S., Cipher, D. J., & Sekscenski, E. (2005). Patient satisfaction with physician assistant, nurse practitioner, and physician care: A national survey of Medicare beneficiaries. *Journal of Clinical and Outcomes Management, 12*(2), 88–92.

Hooker, R., & Freeborn, D. (1995). Patient satisfaction with physician assistant, nurse practitioner, and physician care: a national survey of Medicare beneficiaries. *Journal of Clinical and Outcomes Management, 12*(2), 88–92.

Hooker, R. S., & Muchow, A. N. (2015). Modifying state laws for nurse practitioners and physician assistants can reduce cost of medical services. *Nursing Economics, 33*(2), 88–94.

Horrocks, S., Anderson, E., & Salisbury, C. (2002). Systematic review of whether nurse practitioners working in primary care can provide equivalent care to doctors. *British Medical Journal, 324*(7341), 819–823.

Hunter, L. P., Weber, C. E., Morreale, A. P., & Wall, J. H. (2009). Patient satisfaction with retail health clinic care. *Journal of the American Academy of Nurse Practitioners, 21*(10), 565–570.

Institute of Medicine. (2011). *The future of nursing: Leading change, advancing health.* Retrieved from http://iom.nationalacademies.org/Reports/2010/The-Future-of-Nursing-Leading-Change-Advancing-Health.aspx

Isasi, F., & Krofah, E. (2015). *The expanding role of pharmacists in a transformed health care system.* Washington, DC: National Governors Association Center for Best Practices.

Isetts, B. J., Brummel, A. R., de Oliveira, D. R., & Moen, D. W. (2012). Managing drug-related morbidity and mortality in the patient-centered medical home. *Medical Care, 50*(11), 997–1001.

Japsen, B. (April 23, 2015). Retail clinics hit 10 million annual visits but just 2% of primary care market. *Forbes.* Retrieved from http://www.forbes.com/sites/brucejapsen/2015/04/23/retail-clinics-hit-10-million-annual-visits-but-just-2-of-primary-care-market/

Jennings, N., Clifford, S., Fox, A., O'Connell, J., & Gardner, G. E. (2014). The impact of nurse practitioner services on cost, quality of care, satisfaction and wait times in the emergency department: A systematic review. *International Journal of Nursing Studies, 52*(1), 421–435.

Joint Commission of Pharmacy Practitioners. (2008). *An Action Plan for Implementation of the JCPP Future Vision of Pharmacy Practice.* Washington, DC: Joint Commission of Pharmacy Practitioners. Retrieved from https://pcms.ouhsc.edu/ams/common/docs_oac/ViewOAC_img_blobs.asp?DocID=091276228323

Kleiner, M. M., Marier, A., Park, K. W., & Wing, C. (2014). *Relaxing occupational licensing requirements: Analyzing wages and prices for a medical service.* National Bureau of Economic Research Working Paper 19906. Retrieved from http://www.nber.org/papers/w19906

Kleiner, M. M., & Park, K. W. (2010). *Battles among licensed occupations: Analyzing government regulations on labor market outcomes for dentists and hygienists.* National Bureau of Economic Research Working Paper 16560. Retrieved from http://www.nber.org/papers/w16560

Knapp, D. A., & Knapp, D. E. (2009). Attributes of colleges and schools of pharmacy in the United States. *American Journal of Pharmacy Education, 73*(5), 96.

Knapp, K. K., Paavola, F. G., Maine, L. L., Sorofman, B., & Politzer, R. M. (1998). Availability of primary care providers and pharmacists in the United States. *Journal of the American Pharmaceutical Association, 39*(2), 127–135.

Knapp, K., & Schommer, J. C. (2013). Finding a path through times of change. *American Journal of Pharmacy Education, 77*(5), 91.

Kocher, R. P., & Adashi, E. Y. (2011). Hospital readmissions and the Affordable Care Act: Paying for coordinated quality care. *Journal of the American Medical Association, 306*(16), 1794–1795.

LaBarbera, D. (2004). Physician assistant vocational satisfaction. *Journal of the American Association of Physician Assistants, 17*(10), 34–36, 38–40, 51.

Lewin, G. (2005). Medication therapy management services: A critical review. *Journal of the American Pharmacists Association: Journal of the American Pharmacists Association, 45*(5), 580–587.

Lipton, H. L. (2009). Home is where the health is: Advancing team-based care in chronic disease management. *Archives of Internal Medicine, 169*(21), 1945–1948.

Maine, L. L., Knapp, K. K., & Scheckelhoff, D. J. (2013). Pharmacists and technicians can enhance patient care even more once national policies, practices, and priorities are aligned. *Health Affairs, 32*(11), 1956–1962.

Manolakis, P. G., & Skelton, J. B. (2010). Pharmacists' contributions to primary care in the United States collaborating to address unmet patient care needs: The emerging role for pharmacists to address the shortage of primary care providers. *American Journal of Pharmacy Education, 74*(10), S7.

Martsolf, G. R., Auerbach, D. I., Spetz, J., Pearson, M. L., & Muchow, A. N. (2015). Doctor of nursing practice by 2015: An examination of nursing schools' decisions to offer a doctor of nursing practice degree. *Nursing Outlook, 63*(2), 219–226.

Marvelle, K., & Kraditor, K. (1999). Do PAs in clinical practice find their work satisfying? *Journal of the American Association of Physician Assistants, 12*(11), 43–44, 47, 50.

McGinnis, T., Strand, L. M., & Webb, C. E. (2010). *The patient-centered medical home: Integrating comprehensive medication management to optimize patient outcomes.* Washington, DC: Patient-Centered Primary Care Collaborative.

Mehrotra, A., Liu, H., Adams, J. L., Wang, M. C., Lave, J. R., Thygeson, N. M., . . . McGlynn, E. A. (2009). Comparing costs and quality of care at retail clinics with that of other medical settings for 3 common illnesses. *Annals of Internal Medicine, 151*(5), 321–328.

National Association of Community Health Centers. (2013). *Expanding access to primary care: The role of nurse practitioners, physician assistants, and certified nurse midwives in the health center workforce.* Bethesda, MD: National Association of Community Health Centers. Retrieved from https://www.nachc.com/client/documents/Workforce_FS_0913.pdf

Naylor, M. D., Brooten, D., Campbell, R., Jacobsen, B. S., Mezey, M. D., Pauly, M. V., & Schwartz, J. S. (1999). Comprehensive discharge planning and home follow-up of hospitalized elders: A randomized clinical trial. *Journal of the American Medical Association, 281*(7), 613–620.

Naylor, M. D., Brooten, D. A., Campbell, R. L., Maislin, G., McCauley, K. M., & Schwartz, J. S. (2004). Transitional care of older adults hospitalized with heart failure: A randomized, controlled trial. *Journal of the American Geriatrics Society, 52*(5), 675–684.

Naylor, M. D., & Kurtzman, E. T. (2010). The role of nurse practitioners in reinventing primary care. *Health Affairs, 29*(5), 893–899.

New York Times, The (Editorial). (December 15, 2012). When the doctor is not needed. *The New York Times.* Retrieved from http://www.nytimes.com/2012/12/16/opinion/sunday/when-the-doctor-is-not-needed.html?_r=0.

Newhouse, R. P., Stanik-Hutt, J., White, K. M., Johantgen, M., Bass, E. B., Zangaro, G., Heindel, L. (2011). Advanced practice nurse outcomes 1990-2008: A systematic review. *Nursing Economics, 29*(5), 230–250.

Office of Technology Assessment. (1986). *Nurse Practitioners, Physician Assistants, and Certified Nurse-midwives: An Analysis [Case Study 37].* Washington, DC: US Office of Technology Assessment. Retrieved from http://ota.fas.org/reports/8615.pdf

Owen, J. A., & Burns, A. (2010). Medication use, related problems and medication therapy management. In Truong, H.-A., Bresette, J. L., & Sellers, J. A. (Eds.), *The Pharmacist in Public Health: Education, Applications, and Opportunities.* Washington, DC: American Pharmacists Association.

Petzel, R. (2013). *Utilization of Physician Assistants. Directive 1063.* Washington, DC: Veterans Health Administration.

PricewaterhouseCooper's Health Research Institute. (2014). *Top health industry issues of 2015.* Retrieved from http://www.pwc.com/us/en/health-industries/top-health-industry-issues/index.jhtml.

Ritsema, T. S., Bingenheimer, J. B., Scholting, P., & Cawley, J. F. (2014). Differences in the delivery of health education to patients with chronic disease by provider type, 2005-2009. *Preventing Chronic Disease, 11,* E33.

Romanelli, F., & Tracy, T. S. (2015). A coming disruption in pharmacy? *American Journal of Pharmacy Education, 79*(1), 01.

Safriet, B. J. (1992). *Health care dollars and regulatory sense: The role of advanced practice nursing.* New Haven, CT: Yale University Faculty Scholarship Series. Retrieved from http://digitalcommons.law.yale.edu/fss_papers/4423

Santschi, V., Chiolero, A., Colosimo, A. L., Platt, R. W., Taffé, P., Burnier, M., . . . Paradis, G. (2014). Improving blood pressure control through pharmacist interventions: A meta-analysis of randomized controlled trials. *Journal of the American Heart Association, 3*(2), e000718.

Schneller, E. S. (1978). *The physician's assistant: Innovation in the medical division of labor:* Lexington, MA: Lexington Books.

Schommer, J. C., Cline, R. R., & Larson, T. A. (2005). Pharmacy looks to the future. In Smith, M. I., Fincham, J. E., & Wertheimer A. (Eds), *Pharmacy and the US Health Care System* (pp. 417–443). London: Pharmaceutical Press.

Schommer, J. C., Planas, L. G., & Doucette, W. R. (2015). Establishing pathways for access to pharmacist-provided patient care. *Journal of the American Pharmacists Association, 55*(6), 664–668.

Schommer, J. C., Planas, L. G., Johnson, K. A., Doucette, W. R., Gaither, C. A., Kreling, D. H., & Mott, D. A. (2010). Pharmacist contributions to the US health care system. *Innovations in Pharmacy, 1*(1), 1–16.

Schondelmeyer, S. W. (2009). Recent economic trends in American pharmacy. *Pharmacy in History, 51*(3), 103–126.

Sitkin, S. B. & Sutcliffe, K. M. (1991). Dispensing legitimacy: Professional, organizational, and legal influences on pharmacist behavior. *Research in the Sociology of Organizations, 8,* 269–295.

Smith, M., Bates, D. W., & Bodenheimer, T. (2010). Why pharmacists belong in the medical home. *Health Affairs, 29,* 906–913.

Smith, S. R., & Clancy, C. M. (2006). Medication therapy management programs: Forming a new cornerstone for quality and safety in Medicare. *American Journal of Medical Quality*, *21*(4), 276–279.

Spetz, J., Fraher, E., Li, Y., & Bates, T. (2015). How many nurse practitioners provide primary care? It depends on how you count them. *Medical Care Research and Review*, *72*(3), 359–375.

Spetz, J., Parente, S. T., Town, R. J., & Bazarko, D. (2013). Scope-of-practice laws for nurse practitioners limit cost savings that can be achieved in retail clinics. *Health Affairs*, *32*(11), 1977–1984.

Stange, K. (2014). How does provider supply and regulation influence health care markets? Evidence from nurse practitioners and physician assistants. *Journal of Health Economics*, *33*, 1–27.

Thygeson, M., Van Vorst, K. A., Maciosek, M. V., & Solberg, L. (2008). Use and costs of care in retail clinics versus traditional care sites. *Health Affairs*, *27*(5), 1283–1292.

US Health Resources and Services Administration. (2008). *The adequacy of pharmacist supply: 2004 to 2030.* Rockville, MD: US Health Resources and Services Administration. Retrieved from http://bhpr.hrsa.gov/healthworkforce/pharmacy

US Health Resources and Services Administration. (2013a). *Projecting the supply and demand for primary care practitioners through 2020.* Rockville, MD: US Health Resources and Services Administration.

US Health Resources and Services Administration. (2013b). *The U.S. health workforce chartbook,* Rockville, MD: US Health Resources and Services Administration.

US Health Resources and Services Administration. (2014). *Highlights from the 2012 National Sample Survey of Nurse Practitioners.* Rockville, MD: US Health Resources and Services Administration.

Webb, C. E. (2009). *Integration of pharmacists' clinical services in the patient-centered primary medical home.* Lenexa, KS: American College of Clinical Pharmacy, Retrieved from https://www.accp.com/docs/positions/misc/IntegrationPharmacistClinicalServicesPCMHModel3-09.pdf

Weinick, R. M., Burns, R. M., & Mehrotra, A. (2010). Many emergency department visits could be managed at urgent care centers and retail clinics. *Health Affairs*, *29*(9), 1630–1636.

Willard, R., & Bodenheimer, T. (2012). *The building blocks of high-performing primary care: Lessons from the field.* Oakland, CA: California HealthCare Foundation.

Wittayanukorn, S., Westrick, S. C., Hansen, R. A., Billor, N., Braxton-Lloyd, K., Fox, B. I., & Garza, K. B. (2013). Evaluation of medication therapy management services for patients with cardiovascular disease in a self-insured employer health plan. *Journal of Managed Care Pharmacy*, *19*(5), 385–395.

COMMENTARY TO ACCOMPANY CHAPTER 3

Patricia M. Davidson RN, PhD, FAAN

Dean & Professor
Johns Hopkins School of Nursing
Baltimore.

AS MEDICARE AND MEDICAID MARK their 50th birthday in the United States (U.S.), soaring costs, technological innovation, population aging and the rising burden of chronic disease continue to challenge health care models and the health professions (Altman & Frist, 2015). Skill shortages, cost containment and increasing models of accountability have increased the scrutiny on models of health care delivery from the perspective of payers, consumers and policy makers.

There is likely no point in history where the importance of the configuration of the healthcare workforce has been so important and yet so controversial (Davidson & Du, 2015). Reconfiguring workforce skill mix is a strategy for improving the effectiveness and efficiency of health care. Health care workers are highly controlled by professional and regulatory bodies that are prescriptive of desired knowledge, skills, attitudes, competencies and scope of practice. In the U.S., states have the authority to establish their own regulations regarding licensing and scope of practice of health professions which further contributes to the complexity of articulating workforce models. Spetz and colleagues tackle this complex and multifaceted issue of the healthcare workforce through discussing the history and evolving roles of pharmacists, nurse practitioners (NPs), and physician assistants (PAs). These authors discuss the philosophical genesis of these professional groups and the conceptual basis for their roles in the health care system. Casting the spotlight on issues of power and control and understanding the foundations and development of these professional groups is critical for developing workforce models.

Traditional ways of working in healthcare, have commonly focused on acute and episodic care, and created a fragmented health care system that often meets the needs of health care providers rather than individuals and communities. This approach is challenging traditional models of care as well as educational preparation and credentialing of health care professionals (Davidson, Newton, Tankumpuan, Paull, & Dennison-Himmelfarb, 2015). Traditional, physician centric health care practices are neither affordable, feasible nor sustainable and as a consequence there is a shift in models of collaborative practice and an increasing diversity and heterogeneity in health care providers. These shifts in the workforce composition and also power bases have not been without controversy and manifested in overt turf wars (Iglehart, 2013).

Although pharmacists, NPs, and PAs have both a unique and shared knowledge base and a motivation to improve patient care, there are discrete elements in the origins, development, maturation and role identify of these professional groups, influencing how they engage with patients, health care professionals, institutions, and policy makers. Spetz and colleagues astutely propose that the contributions of pharmacists, NPs, and PAs require generation of: (1) collaborative work systems, (2) information sharing, (3) decision synchronization, (4) incentive alignment, and (5) integrated payment processes within health care systems to improve health care delivery. This reform will require negotiation of patient, provider and health care system factors and coalescing around a common goal of improving health care. Left to their own devices individual professional groups are unlikely to shift but need to be brought together in consortia to address critical health care issues. The Interprofessional Educational Collaboration (IPEC) is an example of such a collaboration. IPEC was formed in 2009 when six national education associations of schools of the health professions formed a collaborative to promote and encourage interprofessional learning experiences (Interprofessional Education Collaborative Expert Panel., 2011). Tailoring and targeting knowledge, skills and competencies to patient needs and desired outcomes is an important start in workforce redesign. Sibbald and colleagues have provided a useful taxonomy to describe workforce roles and functions in skill mix change: enhancement, substitution, delegation and innovation. They also identify that changes in skill mix may also be achieved by altering the boundaries in service delivery through transfer, relocation or liaison (Sibbald, Shen, & McBride, 2004). Considering this nomenclature and also clear documentation of roles as well as scope of practice can be useful in developing, implementing and evaluating workforce models (Krumholz et al., 2006).

The United States Patient Protection and Affordable Care Act, has shifted the focus of healthcare from the individual to the population and through improved coverage increased the number of people accessing care (Kocher & Adashi, 2011). This focus on population based health care and shifts in accountability mean that pharmacists, NPs, and PAs will continue to play a critical role in advancing health care reform. Pressures on the health care system are likely to persist and strategies to improve the quality, access, efficiency and equity are urgently needed. Configuring the health care workforce and skill mix to meet population health care needs is critically important, yet the optimal composition and structure has yet to be defined. Role ambiguity, both within and between professional groups, are barriers to health care reform and are just as important to consider as policy and reimbursement. Changing entrenched beliefs and ways of working will require attention to the educational preparation of health professionals as well as workforce models in industry. Analysis of new approaches to workforce configuration will be required to ensure monitor of quality and outcomes and minimize role ambiguity, redundancies and costs.

References

Altman, D., & Frist, W. H. (2015). Medicare and Medicaid at 50 years: Perspectives of beneficiaries, health care professionals and institutions, and policy makers. *Journal of American Medical Association, 314*(4), 384–395.

Davidson, P. M., & Du, H. (2015). Nurses do not have proprietary rights on caring: but we do on clinical practice models. *Journal of Nursing Management, 23*(4), 409–410.

Davidson, P. M., Newton, P. J., Tankumpuan, T., Paull, G., & Dennison-Himmelfarb, C. (2015). Multidisciplinary management of chronic heart failure: principles and future trends. *Clinical Therapeutics, 37*(10), 2225–2233.

Iglehart, J. K. (2013). Expanding the role of advanced nurse practitioners—risks and rewards. *New England Journal of Medicine, 368*(20), 1935–1941.

Interprofessional Education Collaborative Expert Panel. (2011). *Core competencies for interprofessional collaborative practice: Report of an expert panel*: Interprofessional Education Collaborative Expert Panel. Accessible at https://ipecollaborative.org/About_IPEC.html Retrieved 13th December 2015.

Kocher, R. P., & Adashi, E. Y. (2011). Hospital readmissions and the Affordable Care Act: paying for coordinated quality care. *JAMA, 306*(16), 1794–1795.

Krumholz, H. M., Currie, P. M., Riegel, B., Phillips, C. O., Peterson, E. D., Smith, R., … Faxon, D. P. (2006). A Taxonomy for Disease Management A Scientific Statement From the American Heart Association Disease Management Taxonomy Writing Group. *Circulation, 114*(13), 1432–1445.

Sibbald, B., Shen, J., & McBride, A. (2004). Changing the skill-mix of the health care workforce. *Journal of Health Services Research & Policy, 9*(suppl 1), 28–38.

4

HEALTH PROFESSIONALS AND ORGANIZATIONS—MOVING

TOWARD TRUE SYMBIOSIS

Jeffrey A. Alexander and Gary J. Young

Introduction

Traditionally, hospitals, healthcare systems, and other types of healthcare delivery organizations have been subject to the influence of powerful professional norms from various professional groups on whom these organizations depend to provide patient care. Professional standards and prerogatives have governed what types of personnel are hired, how tasks are distributed among them, and what procedures must be followed in performing these tasks (Nembhard, Alexander, Hoff, & Ramanujam, 2009). As such, a long-standing and important dynamic has existed between healthcare organizations and health professionals that has shaped and will likely continue to shape the way healthcare services are organized and delivered.

However, as a result of various changes in the healthcare sector—increased transparency for quality of care, payment reforms, and new healthcare delivery models—traditional relationships between health professionals and healthcare organizations are being redefined. In this chapter we discuss key developments in the relationship between health professionals and healthcare organizations and the opportunities they offer for improving the efficiency and quality of healthcare services. Much of the extant literature on this topic focuses on relationships between hospitals and physicians as these providers have long been the cornerstone of the US healthcare system. Although we also draw from the US experience with hospital–physician relationships, our analysis and discussion considers relationships between health professionals and healthcare organizations more broadly as they relate to not only hospitals and physicians but other types of health professionals (e.g., nurses, pharmacists) and other types of healthcare organizations (e.g., accountable care organizations, retail clinics). Our analysis of the developments affecting these relationships indicates that healthcare organizations and health professionals will need to work creatively to build organizational models that align their interests and goals, rather than models that are dominated by one group or the other. These models will need to depart from many traditional arrangements and approaches that have characterized relationships between healthcare organizations and health professionals in the past. In this chapter, we outline the broad contours of the types of models that we believe are most viable. The key is for both parties to form and embrace a culture and operating environment that offers shared power and authority as well as flexibility in the types of employment, financial, decision-making, and governance arrangements best supporting the mutual goals and interests of a given healthcare organization and its affiliated health professionals.

The Organization of Professionals in Healthcare Delivery Settings

To examine the relationships between health professionals and healthcare delivery organizations, it is important to understand how professionals have been organized in these settings and the implications for patient care. In contrast to many hierarchical organizations, which are organized and governed along bureaucratic lines with clearly established lines of authority and accountability for all their personnel, the typical healthcare organization has maintained a looser set of administrative linkages with respect to its health professionals. Each group of health professions, whether it be physicians, nurses, pharmacists, or other types of health professionals, has been largely organized within its own unit, where the group's particular professional standards define the clinical roles and responsibilities of unit members. Moreover, few, if any, administrative mechanisms have been in place to bind the various professional groups together for purposes of patient care. These arrangements have been driven by the largely unchallenged professional position that good care is both "individualistic and idiosyncratic," which affords high status to professionals with considerable discretion and freedom from administrative control. As such, health professionals have traditionally operated in what are essentially membership organizations that have had limited formal authority to impose accountability standards on their members or to directly integrate them to achieve organization-wide goals (Freidson, 1984; Alexander & Young, 2010).

The most extreme example of this larger pattern pertains to the hospital–physician relationship. Hospitals have typically operated within a dual hierarchy of control, represented on the one hand by hospital administration and on the other by the physicians comprising the hospital's medical staff. These dual lines of control operate in parallel with each other but rarely have intersected in such a way as to disrupt the relative spheres of influence over issues related to control, resource allocation and professional prerogatives (Young & Saltman, 1985). Although other health professionals such as nurses have also enjoyed some professional prerogatives in hospitals, as hospital employees they have been subject to far more of the traditional oversight and controls common in most hierarchical organizations. Hospitals and other healthcare organizations have maintained very loose control over physicians as a reflection of this professional group's strong professional requirements for autonomy.

Significantly, in contrast to other health professionals, most physicians have typically not been employed directly by hospitals or other healthcare organizations in which they provide patient care but rather have been independent contractors. This type of arrangement has long been in place and, as a reflection of their power, has even given physicians substantial influence over how the resources of healthcare organizations are used. Indeed, the independence of physicians from healthcare organizations has long been a defining feature of the US healthcare industry and one that many commentators point to as an important barrier to improving the efficiency of patient care in organizational settings. (e.g., Pauly & Redisch, 1973; Young & Saltman, 1985; Alexander & Young, 2010).

Moreover, the professional power enjoyed by physicians has also had important implications for their relationships with other professional groups in organizational settings. Despite the recent imperatives for interdisciplinary collaboration for patient care, effective care coordination in healthcare organizations is often missing from professional interactions because of the hierarchical and individualistic culture of medicine (Institute of Medicine [IOM], 2000, 2001; Garman, Leach, & Spector, 2006), which is deeply rooted in the socialization process for health professionals and their institutionalized value systems (Leape & Berwick, 2005). Indeed, the same status characteristics that differentiate the power and prestige individuals hold in broader social contexts also often serve to differentiate status among health professionals within healthcare organizations. Physicians have long had the highest status, power, and autonomy. Other health professionals have historically had a relatively low level of independent authority compared to physicians (e.g., nurses, pharmacists). In organizations such as hospitals, this translates into a clear pecking order where physicians have ultimate authority over other professionals, who essentially serve in a support role for physicians (Starr, 1982; Lichtenstein, Alexander, Wells, & McCarthy, 2004).

It is well understood that the traditional hierarchical culture of healthcare organizations often discourages meaningful collaboration and input, and this places control over patient care in the hands of those often who have the least frequent exposure to patients. For example, many documented accounts exist where a hospital patient was harmed when the attending physician mistakenly ordered the wrong dosage of a medication, and both pharmacist and nurse carried out the order, even though they suspected the error, because of their deference to the physician's authority (Lindeke & Sieckert, 2005; O'Daniel & Rosenstein, 2008). Numerous studies have also demonstrated that more open communication between physicians and nurses in their respective roles as caregivers is associated with lower rates of medication errors and better patient outcomes generally (e.g., Boev & Xia, 2015).

This hierarchy among health professionals also impedes efforts by healthcare organizations to improve coordination of patient care generally by limiting opportunities for redefining roles and responsibilities among health professionals. These roles are often grounded not only in the long-standing professional prerogatives and financial incentives of physicians but also in traditional licensure and accreditation requirements. Such requirements limit the scope of practice of nonphysician health professionals and effectively establish physicians as the ultimate decisionmakers in the management of patient care within organizational settings (IOM, 2003; Federal Trade Commission, 2014; Hain & Fleck, 2014).

The hierarchical patterns of authority, control, and interprofessional relationships described above also extend to patients. The relationship between patients and health professionals has been historically marked by a wide status differential stemming from the professional's specialized knowledge, superior access to health information, and frequently, higher social status (Freidson, 1970; Brody, 1980). A patient was expected to behave passively, interacting with professionals in a cooperative, trustful, and compliant manner (Beisecker & Beisecker, 1993). These roles were accepted, and even considered desirable, under the assumption that maximizing professional control over treatment optimizes health outcomes (Charles, Whelan, & Gafni, 1999; Truog, 2012). As discussed in Chapter 1, patients in recent years have become much more engaged in their care, a development that serves to reduce status differentials between health professionals and patients.

In sum, traditional relationships between health professionals and healthcare organizations have been characterized by the autonomy of professional groups with regard to their patient care practices, the high level of independence and status afforded to physicians, and the relatively passive role of patients in terms of their encounters with health professionals.

New Demands on Healthcare Organizations and Health Professionals

Escalating demands for greater efficiency and higher quality have resulted in both new organizational arrangements and management practices (Guterman, Davis, Stremikis, & Drake, 2010). In terms of organizational arrangements, hospitals and other types of healthcare providers have been aggressively consolidating into complex health systems, including accountable care organizations [ACOs], which often shift the locus of governance away from local communities to centralized corporate entities (Alexander, Morlock, & Gifford, 1988; Young, Desai, & Hellinger, 2000; Bazzoli, 2004; Alexander, Young, Weiner, & Hearld, 2009). Healthcare organizations are also adopting various management practices such as clinical guidelines, provider profiling, and care management procedures as an attempt to exert some control over how health professionals use resources for managing patient care (e.g., Casalino et al., 2013; McConnel, Lindrooth, Wholey, & Bloom, 2013).

As healthcare organizations undergo these changes to adapt to growing pressures for efficiency, quality, and patient-centered care, key questions are raised regarding the viability of traditional relationships between health professionals and healthcare organizations. Specifically, will traditional relationships persist, and, if not, how might they need to change in an evolving healthcare landscape? Given prevailing developments and trends in US healthcare, traditional professional–organizational relationships are no longer likely to be viable and must be fundamentally redefined. In particular, the high degree of specialization and autonomy of the health professions within healthcare organizations has been identified as a major barrier to improving the coordination and continuity of patient care (Garman et al., 2006; Nembhard et al., 2009). Although few would dispute that the knowledge and skills of individual health professions are important for high-quality care, increasingly health professionals are being asked to practice collaboratively within well-defined patient care teams and larger practice arrangements. In these settings, the quality of care delivered by professionals depends critically on the functioning of the system in preventing errors; coordinating care among settings and different types of professionals; and ensuring that relevant, accurate information is available when needed. The traditional individualistic approach to patient care practiced by many physicians and other healthcare professionals is not well suited to promoting collective responsibility for patient care quality, operational efficiency, or other areas of performance. This lack of integration has been reinforced by turf battles among groups of professionals (e.g., physicians and nurses) as each one struggles to expand its professional practice domain or, alternatively, protect its control over its professional prerogatives.

Perhaps the most problematic aspect for achieving better clinical integration within healthcare organizations is the poor alignment of incentives and strategic goals between the various professional groups and the organizations that use their services. Healthcare delivery organizations historically have sought to engage in strategic relations with professionals to accomplish a limited set of objectives: (a) protect against threat of agency from professionals who have traditionally borne little financial risk for the care of patients; (b) reduce transaction costs by developing economies of scale and integrating professionals into the structure of the delivery organization; (c) achieve market power both upstream and downstream over suppliers and customers, respectively; and (d) develop capabilities that differentiate organizations from competitors in the areas of innovation, technology, and quality (Rundall, Alexander, & Shortell, 2005; Alexander & Young, 2010). Professionals and organizations have pursued these objectives narrowly so as to maximize their own distinct financial interests and goals with little consideration for how best to meet the needs and preference of patients while delivering high-quality, cost-effective care.

In theory, stronger alignment of incentives and goals between healthcare organizations and health professionals will result in more strategically responsive organizations that can deliver cost-effective, patient-centered care (Burns, Andersen, & Shortell, 1990; Burns, Shortell, & Andersen, 1998). Alignment enables professionals and organizations to act in concert rather than at cross-purposes and, with optimal effort, to achieve important but challenging strategic objectives. However, the alignment of financial and strategic interests among organizations and professionals can be difficult, given differences that exist between the two entities with respect to economic incentives and patient care orientation (Dukerich, Golden, & Shortell, 2002). Healthcare organizations face the challenge of developing policies, structures, and incentives to improve quality within a domain that has traditionally been the province of highly autonomous professionals. Indeed, a major impasse for organizational–professional alignment has been the position of many professionals that they serve as the last line of defense against poor quality of care. This attitude reinforces the perspective that quality of care stems from the individual provider's relationship with the individual patient and that attempts to oversee and standardize care processes should be resisted.

At the same time, attempts to better integrate and align the interests between organizations and health professionals are being met with new challenges as some types of health professionals (e.g., nurse practitioners, physical therapists) are gaining more opportunities to be liberated from the hospital and other types of healthcare organizations. As noted in Chapter 1, this is occurring through changes in scope of practice laws and payment policies that in effect give some health professionals more independence from healthcare organizations than they have had in the past. As such, healthcare organizations that seek to recruit and retain such professionals may need to be much more attentive than they have had to be in the past to the concerns and interests of these professionals. That said, the dynamics of these relationships will also likely depend at least in part on the supply of and demand for the services of a given type of health professional.

Adding to these issues are the emerging conflicts within healthcare organizations that are emanating from blurring professional boundaries for physicians, nurse practitioners, and other professionals such as pharmacists. As different professions compete for resources and influence within healthcare organizations, these organizations are under greater pressure to integrate different professionals into teams and promote interdisciplinary collaboration. Healthcare organizations face the challenge of trying to reconcile these conflicts while integrating different professions into coherent provider teams. As noted in Chapter 1, the growing literature on ACOs, which are designed to integrate different types of health professionals for patient care, indicates that these organizations are faced with growing and possibly competing pressures from different professional groups seeking to enhance their roles in these organizations (e.g., Smith, Bates, & Bodenheimer, 2013; Dupree et al., 2014).

Learning from the Past—What Has and Has Not Worked, and Why?

The need to align the interests and behaviors of healthcare organizations and health professionals is receiving increased attention because of the factors outlined earlier in this chapter and in Chapter 1. However, the issue of alignment is hardly new. Past attempts to integrate and align healthcare organizations and health professionals have not always rationalized the delivery of healthcare, but instead have made it more complex and contentious. It is important to learn from these efforts for the purpose of designing organizational systems that truly create a symbiosis between organizations and professionals. An overriding lesson from the past is that effective alignment between healthcare organizations and health professionals cannot be solved solely through traditional administrative arrangements.

Many previous efforts at alignment occurred during the "managed care" era in the late 1980s and 1990s, when healthcare providers were under pressure from payers to contain costs and better coordinate care. Hospitals in particular undertook numerous initiatives to exert more control over their health professionals. In the case of physicians, these initiatives took various forms, including acquiring physician practices, placing practicing physicians on governing boards, creating physician–hospital joint ventures such as physician–hospital organizations (PHOs), and introducing risk-sharing schemes emphasizing both individual and organization-wide performance goals (Morrisey, Alexander, Burns, & Johnson, 1996; Alexander et al., 2001). Few of these initiatives, however, proved to be effective either in terms of improved performance, greater loyalty, or identification of physicians with their organizations.

At base, these initiatives were founded on a simplistic and ultimately faulty assumption—that by subjecting physicians to some measure of external control, regulating the conditions of employment, and replacing the loose collegial form of organization with administrative hierarchy, physicians would conform to organizational goals and align their behavior more with managerial goals. In so doing, physicians would become "tied to the organization" and thus likelier to identify with it and its imperatives (Burns, Andersen, & Shortell, 1990; Burns, Shortell, & Andersen, 1998). This proved not to be the case, as many hospitals ultimately abandoned their initiatives to employ or otherwise integrate physicians through practice acquisitions after experiencing significant financial losses from these initiatives. (These losses, according to some estimates, often exceeded $100,000 for each employed physician [e.g., Kocher & Sahni, 2011].)

Past efforts by hospitals to align other types of professionals also proved problematic, even for professional groups whose members have traditionally been employees of healthcare organizations. For example, as a tactic to adapt to managed care pressures, many hospital administrators sought greater oversight over clinical departments such as nursing and pharmacy to reduce costs and gain flexibility in delivering patient care services. Hospital administrators often sought to reduce or otherwise oversee staffing levels of these departments through centralized personnel controls. Some hospitals also adopted organizational structures that either completely or partially dismantled such departments in favor of distinct clinical service lines that brought various health professionals together under a single point of decision-making authority (Charns & Tewksbury, 1993; Parker, Charns, & Young, 2001; Young, Charns, & Hereen, 2004). These initiatives have often been a source of significant strain between affected health professionals and administrators (e.g., Charns & Tewksbury, 1993; Weinberg, 2003).

Accordingly, purely formal administrative arrangements, whether through employment, shared financial risk models, or centralized management structures, have generally not been sufficient to fully align the interests of professionals and healthcare organizations. However, as noted, external pressures for greater alignment between professionals and healthcare organizations continue to increase in ways that neither party can ignore without placing itself in financial jeopardy. Some research indicates that when health professionals identify (i.e., experience a sense of oneness) much more closely with their own profession than the organization with which they are affiliated, they will be much less inclined to pursue organization-wide goals even when it is contrary to their financial interests (Hekman, Bigley, Steensma, &

Hereford, 2009). Accordingly, greater alignment between professionals and organizations likely requires professionals to identify more closely with the organizations to which they are affiliated. As such, we next consider ways to conceptualize the changing nature of relationships between health professionals and healthcare organizations. We then propose recommendations for breaking through long-standing barriers to their effective alignment.

Conceptual Framework for Redefining Relationships between Healthcare Organizations and Health Professionals

Previous attempts to integrate and align professionals and organizations have frequently met with difficulty because they have directly conflicted with the cultural norms of health professionals by subordinating these groups to an administrative hierarchy without attention to their own concerns and values. As noted, many healthcare organizations have sought to unilaterally constrain the autonomy of professionals (although not completely) through the imposition of administrative controls. Such initiatives can be examined from the standpoint of Scott's general classification of professional–organizational structures: autonomous professional, heteronomous, and conjoint (Scott, 1982; Scott & Davis, 2007). Whereas in autonomous professional structures, organizations defer substantially to the professional prerogatives of their professional members, heteronomous structures are characterized by the imposition of administrative controls on professionals. Conjoint structures, which we discuss later on in this chapter, are intended to achieve a balance between administrative and professional prerogatives and values.

From the standpoint of the Scott framework, hospitals and other types of healthcare organizations have made various attempts to transition from autonomous professional structures to heteronomous ones relative to health professionals. In such structures, professional autonomy in the treatment of individual patients (micro care) is limited in favor of a well-defined division of labor combined with managerial oversight to achieve coordination and control of professionals' individual contributions. Significant efforts are expended to codify and standardize clinical processes to promote improvements in professional practice, greater consistency among professionals, and maximize outcomes for populations of patients (macro care). As noted, efforts by healthcare organizations to move physicians from autonomous to heteronomous structures have generally not been successful in the past. Furthermore, although most other types of health professionals such as nurses and pharmacists have long operated under some level of administrative controls within healthcare organizations (and thus have performed their work within structures that were closer to heteronomous structures), these groups have also resisted efforts to impose additional controls on their patient care activities.

Still, the previously discussed external pressures on US healthcare organizations for better performance may well prove to be key forces for redefining relationships between healthcare organizations and professionals. Under new methods of provider compensation for physicians and healthcare organizations, including hospitals and ACOs (e.g., global payment, bundled payments), both parties assume some level of financial risk-sharing for their performance relative to quality and efficiency metrics (Fisher, Staiger, Bynum, & Gottlieb, 2006). In principle, such risk-sharing promotes collaboration between healthcare organizations and physicians specifically because high utilization and costs will result in financial deficits for both types of providers. In practice, the physician group's form of compensation, incentives, and governance buffer these effects. For example, the incentives inherent in financial risk-sharing can be lost if individual physician compensation is not strongly linked to holding costs below the group's budget target.

Moreover, as healthcare organizations seek to adapt to payment reform and other pressures for performance accountability, they need to be concerned about their relationships with all the professional groups with whom they depend for patient care. As noted, to perform at a high level of quality and efficiency, it is expected that healthcare organizations must be able to break down the long-standing silos that have existed among the various professional groups for purposes of better coordination of patient care. Healthcare organizations face the challenge of developing policies, procedures, and incentives to improve quality within a domain that has traditionally been the province of highly autonomous professionals. The primary concern of these professions has been with their own individual performance, not the overall performance of the organization with which they are affiliated. Given these developments and the disappointing experiences from previous attempts to align and integrate professionals and organizations, a significant shift to heteronomous structures is by no means a given for physicians or other types of health professionals. Rather, both a hybridization and diversity of organizational–professional relations are likely to emerge, which reflect a synthesis or accommodation of both professional and managerial perspectives.

Conjoint Models of Organization—Beyond Professional or Managerial Dominance

These emergent organizational arrangements may be described as conjoint structures, which are characterized by roughly equal power of professional participants and administrators, and equal importance of their functions. Instead of domination by one group (as with the traditional professional or heteronomous structures), coexistence in a state of interdependence and mutual influence and multiple centers of power is not uncommon (Scott, 1982; Kitchener, Caronna, & Shortell, 2005). The recognition of the presence and the legitimacy of both micro care and macro care and the tensions these perspectives engender are features that distinguish the conjoint structure from the previously discussed arrangements for linking healthcare organizations and health professionals.

The principles underlying the conjoint approach to integrating and aligning professional and organizational interests have profound implications for the organizational arrangements in healthcare. For example, we expect to see an increase in loosely aligned organizational arrangements that reflect the diverse and sometimes conflicting interests of administrators and professionals. These have begun to take form in organizations such as ACOs where hospitals and physician groups, for example, are bound by a common strategic/reimbursement framework but not necessarily tied together under common ownership or other formal administrative arrangements. Similarly, the growth and enhanced professional prerogatives of other professions such as nurse practitioners may free them from the constraints of working under the supervision of physicians, thus increasing their ability to negotiate with healthcare organizations on the terms of their employment as well as scope of practice.

These structures increase the flexibility of both healthcare organizations and professional groups to align with others that share their goals and practice values as well as presenting greater choice regarding what administrative structures would work best for achieving strategic goals. For example, healthcare organizations may increasingly approach relationships with health professionals from a "make or buy" perspective—that is, engaging with professionals on the open market for their services under contract or tying them more closely to the organization through formal employment arrangements. As such, healthcare organizations are likely to begin examining the transaction costs of contracting with health professions who traditionally have been their employees.

This flexibility will likely spawn greater diversity of organizational arrangements than in the past. For example, in settings where professionals have been successful in influencing regulation that supports traditional professional practices and professional control, or where they are more active in wielding market power and resources, we might expect more loosely structured arrangements between them and healthcare organizations. These arrangements are not well suited for dictating specific clinical protocols or care management procedures to professionals. As such, in these settings, healthcare organizations will need to be creative to adapt to new payment policies, increased competition, or other changes in their operating environment as they arise (Nelson et al., 2002). That is, with limited recourse to managerial controls, healthcare organizations will need to be that much more focused on building alignment between themselves and their affiliated health professionals on the basis of a strong shared culture for patient care. For example, healthcare organizations that seek to motivate providers to pursue certain performance outcomes will need to engage providers so that they see these outcomes as important and consistent with their own professional values.

Given that some level of conflict is both expected and integral to conjoint structures, we also expect to see the emergence of interdependent structures that allow the conflicting parties to come together to express and deal with their differences. These might take the form of joint operating committees, shared governance, or matrix structures that combine professional and administrative components to develop strategies to accommodate both macro and micro care priorities for patient care. For example, quality assurance programs that often consist of a set of diverse and uncoordinated medical staff committees need to be gathered into organized units that support the involvement of all types of health professionals (and healthcare managers) for purposes of data collection and analysis. Regardless of the form these interdependent structures assume, their participants must acknowledge the legitimacy of each other's goals and be willing to use the available decision-making structures and processes to develop creative, less bureaucratic solutions to pressing healthcare needs.

From this type of model, we can expect health professionals to be more likely to develop a strong identification with their affiliated healthcare organizations. But identification will never be a given. So from a recruitment standpoint, healthcare organizations will also need to consider the characteristics of health professionals such as personality or career goals that make them a good fit for their organizations. Currently, little systematic research offers guidance to healthcare organizations on this point. We know in a general sense that certain types of physicians are attracted to integrated systems such as the Mayo Clinic and Kaiser Permanente, but little is known about how to identify and match characteristics of health professionals with the culture and structure of a given healthcare organization. Accordingly, conjoint structures may be most appropriate for developing the type of health professional–healthcare organization relationships that are required for environments that emphasize global payment, accountability for quality-related performance goals including population health outcomes, and patient-centered care. At a broad level, these models will emphasize flexibility in employment and financial arrangements between an organization and its affiliated health professionals. It will also comprise management systems that tolerate and are capable of resolving some level of conflict between the interests of the organization and its health professionals. In the following section, we discuss specific components for making a conjoint model work in healthcare organizations.

Making New Conjoint Structures Work

We have argued that conjoint structures for accommodating patient care issues are likely to be more common as some professional groups gain greater independence and others organize in ways to assume collective responsibility for care. Given the powerful cultural norms that characterize most professional groups, it is highly questionable whether structural solutions to achieving greater alignment between professionals and healthcare organizations can be completely effective by themselves. The success of conjoint forms of organizations will likely depend on the specific supporting elements of these arrangements that extend beyond structural arrangements. Although, not exhaustive, we discuss below several features of conjoint organizational arrangements that may enhance their effectiveness.

The first feature is shared governance. Beyond their structural features, conjoint organizational arrangements require participating healthcare organizations and professions to make decisions about the governance and management of the entity, the criteria for selecting professional members, and the rules for sharing financial risk and profits (Hosler & Nadle, 2000). Traditional organizational structures and financial incentives have impeded the ability of both healthcare organization governing boards and professional groups to respond to these pressures. Shared governance implies policy making and oversight over the entire enterprise, not just its individual components. It also implies inclusion and equal power and influence among all professional and administrative groups. In addition, it incorporates shared decision-making arrangements that are closer to the front lines of patient care. A recently published literature review of the effects of governance mechanisms on health workforce outcomes revealed shared governance was consistently associated with such outcomes as job satisfaction and interprofessional collaboration (Hastings, Armitrage, Mallinson, Jackson, & Suter, 2014).

The second essential component of a successful conjoint approach to organizational–professional relations is a robust information system. Because decisions in conjoint organizations must transcend entrenched professional and administrative interests, timely data that reflect agreed on performance standards and operational requirements are essential for developing a common language and engendering trust among participating professional groups and delivery organizations. Without such data-based transparency and decision-making, the tensions inherent in conjoint forms of organization are likely to provoke conflict rather than foster creative solutions. Healthcare experts have pointed to information systems as a central requirement for developing successful ACOs (Agency for Healthcare Research and Quality, 2014).

The third component of successful conjoint arrangements is team-based care. Specialized care delivered through fragmented and rigid clinical units is inconsistent with changing payment policies designed to reward coordinated care within and across organizational boundaries. Furthermore, such fragmented care is also inconsistent with the current emphasis on patient-centered care, where patients are ongoing partners in their care and not simply raw material to be worked on in episodic fashion. Team-based care enables members to coordinate care and to bring diverse clinical orientations and skill sets to the diagnosis and treatment of patients. It also affords the patient some measure of participation in care decisions by establishing shared goals that reflect patient and family priorities (Aucott et al., 1995).

To promote full commitment by all professional members, treatment teams should assume a relatively flat authority structure and promote participative decision-making. Ideally, while conducting team business, teams should suspend at least to some degree authority relationships that exist in other settings so that the exchange of information is free flowing and unencumbered by traditional patterns of interaction (e.g., Grumbach & Bodenheimer, 2004; Van Der Vegt & Bunderson, 2005). Team-based care stands in marked contrast to the hierarchical work relations in most traditional care delivery organizations, which, as noted, have accorded the physician a role of almost absolute autonomy and control over patient care processes. Although in concept, team-based care is a critical component for building alignment between healthcare organizations and affiliated health professionals, the evidence also indicates that forming successful patient care teams over extended periods of time is challenging. Little evidence exists addressing the best way to form and manage teams to produce better patient outcomes. Thus, healthcare organizations and health professionals must be prepared for a significant investment in time and resources to experiment with different approaches to team-based care (e.g., Grumbach & Bodenheimer, 2004; Lemieux-Charles & McGuire, 2006).

In conjoint structures, true team-based care is supported by expanding scopes of practices of professional groups such as nurses and pharmacists. For example, nurses and other ancillary professionals have advocated a form of collaboration with physicians where the nonphysicians have primary responsibility for health maintenance, prevention, and diagnosis and treatment of routine cases, while the physicians retain responsibility for the diagnosis and treatment of complex cases and the prescription of medications (e.g., Cassidy, 2012; Everett et al., 2013). Although in many states, this type of division of labor between physicians and nurses is not in line with current scopes of practice and professional norms, as has been discussed elsewhere in this book, there is some momentum to modify these rules to give nonphysician health professionals greater power and control in patient care decision-making. In this vein, some healthcare organizations may be inclined to support expanded scopes of practice for nurse practitioners, pharmacists, and other types of health professionals as a tactic for integrating these professionals into effective patient care delivery teams. At the same time, expanding scopes of practices provide some health professionals with greater opportunities to form their own practices and compete with the healthcare organizations that have traditionally employed them. Expanding scopes of practice may also create significant managerial challenges for healthcare organizations due to the turf battles that can ensue among health professionals from changing and overlapping boundaries for their clinical roles in patient care (e.g., Gardner, 2010). In addition, healthcare organizations should carefully consider how important employment of health professionals is to the development of team-based care as part of their "make-or-buy decisions" for such personnel that, as we previously noted, may become increasingly common.

A fourth condition for promoting successful conjoint organizational arrangements is an appropriately designed system for incentives and risk-sharing. As noted, payment reform in the United States may well prove to be a key force for redefining relationships between healthcare organizations and professionals. However, financial incentives created by risk-sharing between health professionals and healthcare organizations are effective only under certain conditions. Several authors have recognized that the effects of such payment mechanisms may partially depend on organizational factors such as type of governance, professional leadership, information dissemination, and organizational culture, discussed elsewhere in this chapter (Kralewski et al., 2000, Alexander et al., 2001). For example, if health professionals believe they have no say in the formulation of incentives in compensation systems, they may be less willing to abide by them. This suggests that physicians and other health professionals must be accorded a measure of "soft autonomy" in shaping the direction of the delivery organization (Levay & Waks, 2009). Recent research demonstrates that health professionals respond much more significantly to performance-based incentive systems within healthcare organizations when the performance measures match their own patient care values and goals (Young, Beckman, & Baker, 2012). The challenge in creating such risk-sharing is establishing the appropriate balance between macro care and micro care priorities and ensuring that the resultant system of incentives reflects the goals of the system as opposed to those of any particular constituency or interest group.

Perhaps the most important and challenging aspect of forming successful conjoint organizational–professional arrangements is creating a common culture that binds different professional groups and, frequently, different organizations through a commonly held set of values and beliefs. Some commentators raise important questions about the prospects of alignment between healthcare organizations and professionals, particularly physicians (IOM & National Academy of Engineering, 2011). They contend that the cultures of physicians and physician groups represent a poor fit with the strategy of forming organizational linkages to truly bind physicians to healthcare organizations. This has been expressed most often when administratively dominated approaches such as formal governance and administrative arrangements have inhibited professional autonomy or subjected professionals to administrative controls removed from the actual delivery of patient care. Violation of these cultural norms may actually decrease physicians' feelings of identity and alignment with the system (Dukerich et al., 2002).

Similarly, efforts by healthcare organizations to exert greater control over other types of health professionals may also encounter resistance from those professionals. To move forward, healthcare organizations need to develop a culture that can meet their operational needs but also support the professional interests and concerns of the individuals on whose clinical expertise they depend for excellent patient care. Some delivery organizations, for example, have attempted to foster what they refer to as a culture of ownership (e.g., Tye, 2012; Sullivan, 2014). In such a culture all members of the organization, regardless of their professional affiliation or departmental home, are encouraged to take a vested, personal stake in the outcomes their patient experience and in the means to do what it takes to make improvements. To promote this type of culture, delivery organizations appear to create opportunities for health professions to access detailed results of the organization's financial and clinical performance and offer support to those who require assistance to understand the information. In addition, they form multiple types of advisory committees so that health professionals have a diverse set of opportunities to voice their perspectives about how the organization is managed to key decision makers. These organizations may also create self-managed teams to replace or at least supplement traditional departments.

Such a culture stands in marked contrast to a heteronomous arrangement where professionals perform according to a narrowly defined job description, contractual obligation, or norms of their professional group but do not assume responsibility for the broader goals of the organization. Even if professionals lose certain forms of work autonomy through standardization of guidelines and protocols, affording them "soft" autonomy in matters related to their cultural values may prove important. Although no empirical studies claim to examine the performance effects for healthcare organizations from an ownership culture specifically, many studies have systematically examined the performance effects of related cultural attributes such as participative decision-making arrangements for health professionals and consistent recognition of the organization's mission to provide excellent patient care (e.g., Taylor, Clay-Williams, Hogden, Braithwaite, & Groene, 2015). The evidence from these studies appears generally to support the positive impact of these cultural attributes on quality of care.

Examples from Practice

The movement toward conjoint organizational–professional arrangements is still in the emergent stages as health delivery organizations and professional groups seek to redefine their roles in the new healthcare environment. How they will have an impact on quality and costs has yet to be determined by researchers. However, selective examples from practice may illustrate how these organizational arrangements can be made operational and successful. We focus on three areas that highlight what we believe are important principles of conjoint models for professional–organizational arrangements—shared governance, information technology, and team-based patient care.

The first example involves shared governance. This is a fundamental cornerstone of conjoint arrangements because it binds different power centers into a coherent common enterprise. Advocate Health Care, a large healthcare system in Chicago, is a joint venture between physicians in various practices including solo and group, single-specialty and multispecialty, employed and independent physicians (Shields, Patel, Manning, & Sacks, 2011). The partnership's independent physicians share in the governance of Advocate Health Care. This is accomplished through two equal classes of governance votes, one for Advocate and one for local PHOs. The votes of a majority of each class are required for a measure to pass. Physicians elect the leaders of each local PHO, who then send a delegate to the overall partnership board.

In addition, employed physicians occupy many of the Advocate governance seats in the partnership, which means that physicians are in a strong position vis à vis hospital managers to influence decisions affecting the partnership. This arrangement creates a structure that enables physicians and hospitals to collaborate to improve care with common quality and cost effectiveness goals. Physicians and hospitals are collectively accountable for quality and cost during negotiations with payers because the partnership negotiates on behalf of both Advocate and physicians and signs contracts that apply to both parties. The Advocate governance system is complex but effectively addresses the need for decision-making at different levels of the organization and with different classes of professionals. It also highlights the importance of shared governance by giving professionals, in this case physicians, a strong voice in system decision-making rather than a more token role.

A second example illustrates the importance of information technology in conjoint organizational–professional arrangements. HealthCare Partners, a large California-based medical group, is committed to developing a sophisticated health information technology (HIT) infrastructure that connects all stakeholders in the network: administrators, medical group and independent practice association providers, and patients. As part of this effort, HealthCare Partners has spent considerable time developing tools for end users (e.g., managers, medical group site leaders, regional directors, and patients). Its resource center collects, aggregates, and further standardizes the information, and it provides automated, comprehensive reports on HealthCare Partners' financial, quality, and operational performance. A sophisticated internal data warehouse aggregates and harmonizes clinical, administrative, and financial data. The data warehouse pulls information from disparate electronic health records and other sources (including patient portals) into a standardized format, giving HealthCare Partners a well-rounded view of its patients and enabling it to identify high-risk and high-cost patients. HealthCare Partners' HIT infrastructure and data warehouse serve as the foundation on which it can design care coordination tools and programs (Gbemudu et al., 2012). Its approach to information is based on pursuing a common foundation of agreed on metrics and tools that can be used by multiple stakeholders in the system to engage in problem-solving, resource allocation decisions, and strategic planning, even if the administrative and professional groups are organizationally distinct. Importantly, this approach also can give patients access to information that helps them become better decision makers and partners in their care. Finally, such a common information system promotes a culture of ownership in the system by identifying and rewarding positive individual performance.

A third example is team-based care. Team-based patient care has been defined as "the provision of comprehensive health services by at least two health professionals who work collaboratively along with patients, family caregivers, and community service providers on shared goals within and across settings to achieve care that is safe, effective, patient-centered, timely, efficient, and equitable" (Mitchell et al., 2012, p. 5). The need for team-based care arises in part from a growing body of evidence suggesting that individuals coping with multiple chronic conditions are particularly vulnerable to coordination and communications breakdowns in care. Addressing such issues is particularly important in conjoint arrangements where multiple care sites and provider groups are potentially involved. However, as noted, the literature indicates that developing successful patient care teams is very challenging as many studies report disappointing results from team-based interventions to improve patient care.

Institutions such as the University of Pennsylvania are striving to meet this challenge through a transitional care model of team care, which incorporates organizational units such as hospitals, primary care practices, home healthcare, and hospice (Mitchell et al., 2012). The model depends on a team of providers comprised of a transitional care nurse (TCN) and other health professionals (e.g., physicians, social workers, physical therapists, hospice staff, home health aides) who collaboratively identify, plan, and execute a plan of care for high-risk patients. Team members identify older adults with multiple chronic conditions and two or more risk factors via a standardized screening assessment and risk criteria tool. The patient is then paired with a TCN, who initiates a collaborative, comprehensive assessment of the patient's health status and simultaneously develops a care plan with the patient and family caregivers to address their identified goals. The care plan is continually reevaluated by the team to ensure it meets the needs and preferences of the patient and family caregivers. To make transitional care models work, the organization provides time, space, and support for meaningful, comprehensive information exchange between and among team members, particularly when a new team forms—for example, when a new patient and family begins to work with the team. The organization also facilitates the establishment and maintenance of a written plan of care that is accessible and updatable by all team members and supports the team's capacity to monitor progress toward shared goals for the patient, family, and team. Research is needed to fully evaluate the impact of this model on patient outcomes. However, this and other team models do hold promise for building more effective relationships between healthcare organizations and health professionals.

Implications for Research and Practice

Future efforts to align healthcare organizations and health professions will have important implications for research and practice. Given the lack of success in aligning professional and organizational interests in the past, using similar integration approaches in today's healthcare environment may not realize the desired aims. In particular, past experience has taught us that it is exceedingly difficult to achieve alignment, given the cultural separation between delivery organizations and many professional groups and the mistrust that often characterizes their relationships. For example, health maintenance organizations (HMOs) that acquired physician clinics or developed staff models, including Cigna, Aetna, and FHP International, found they could not manage medical practices successfully (e.g., Levick, 1995; Jurgeleit, 1997; Butcher, 2008). Consequently, they spun off these organizations to physician practice management companies that claimed to have expertise in this area. Indeed, professional–organizational arrangements have often been proposed, developed, and then underutilized or even undone, particularly when one side is dominant in the arrangement based on decision-making authority.

From this perspective, organizations should consider more contractual linkages that bring the parties together on key enterprises but otherwise leave each with the autonomy to manage their own activities. Even among HMOs where integration of hospital and physicians have had long-standing histories, the most common models are not single-firm entities, but contractual arrangements of groups and network models. However, it is also evident that organizations and professionals are using a variety of new integration strategies rather than ones based exclusively on contractual networks. The presence of multiple integration approaches under the broad heading of conjoint arrangement may suggest that no one strategy works best or is appropriate for all organizations or professional groups. Organizations are experimenting with different approaches to integration as a way of dealing with uncertainly and to accommodate different cohorts of professionals with different levels of readiness for integration. For example, although a trend once again exists among hospitals and health systems to employ physicians, some delivery organizations are choosing as an alternative to integrate physicians through so-called comanagement arrangements, which are strategic alliances that give physicians financial incentives to assume managerial and fiscal responsibility for distinct clinical activities (e.g., Dowell, 2010). The variety of professional–organizational integration approaches currently being tried under the ACO initiative also underscores the fact that integration requires the participation of both organizations and professional groups. It cannot be unilaterally imposed. Clearly, new payment schemes may affect one party more than another, or one party may have more alternatives than another, when these macro changes become a force in the market. Both conditions may preclude universal, unilateral responses by organizations and professionals.

Accordingly, important research opportunities exist to examine which specific arrangements, financial incentives, and related management practices work best under which conditions including market competition, payment policies, and clinical needs of patients. For example, under what circumstances is it most effective to contract for the services of certain types of health professionals than employ them directly? Under contractual models, what systems and practices are effective for ensuring that professionals are appropriately accountable for their performance and committed to the organization? What are best practices for forming and managing patient care teams?

Of course, it remains to be seen whether loosely structured arrangements and power sharing can be sustained without the coherence, trust, and loyalty that characterizes more tightly integrated arrangements. If greater power sharing, more contractual arrangements, and increased conflict will characterize organizational–professional relations in the future, what will bind these organizations and professionals together in a common mission? Although it may seem that professional identification precludes the strong organizational identification needed for successful integration in healthcare, this does not have to be the case. At the Mayo Clinic, the workforce has embraced both professional and organizational identities since the clinic's founding in the late 1800s. Many attribute this to its founders who instilled a core value that has always resonated with the workforce: the needs of the patient come first (Viggiano, Pawlina, Lindor, Olsen, & Cortese, 2007). However, legacy is not the only means to strong organizational identification.

Management research has identified at least two practice-related strategies for fostering the organizational identification needed for integration of organizational and professional interests: (1) increase the attractiveness of the perceived organizational identity, and (2) increase the attractiveness of the construed external image (i.e., the image held by those outside of the organization) (Dukerich et al., 2002). The former strategy builds on the finding that physicians feel stronger organizational identification where they perceive alignment between their goals and values and those of the organization. The second strategy reflects the finding that physicians' feelings about organizations with which they are affiliated is influenced by how outsiders view those organizations. Thus, the challenge for delivery organizations is to find ways to highlight the similarities between professional and organizational values and showcase their positive attributes (e.g., pro bono work, awards, new facilities) to enhance their external image. For example, although professionals typically focus on micro care oriented to the care of individuals and organizations focus on macro care oriented on the well-being of populations, both are likely to believe in the superordinate goals of improving quality of care and patient satisfaction. But as previously noted, research is needed to guide healthcare organizations about how best to recruit health professionals so that a strong fit exists between the organization and the professional.

Finally, much of what makes the conjoint approach to organizational–professional arrangements work depends on process-related factors such as power sharing, conflict resolution, and shared governance rather than structural drivers. Despite the importance of these process-related factors, structural characteristics tend to dominate the research literature. To the extent that these process-related factors are, in fact, important drivers of cost and quality in conjoint arrangements, researchers may wish to complement the traditional focus on large samples and structural correlates of outcomes with intensive, qualitative research on management and governance processes conducted in smaller samples of organizations. Researchers should also consider how process research being done in other sectors can be adapted and applied in a healthcare context. For example, human resource management studies in the general management sector have resulted in a sophisticated, practical understanding of how to recruit, retain, and deploy staff effectively.

Conclusions

In this chapter we have attempted to make the case that in a changing healthcare environment characterized by greater accountability, financial risk, patient voice, and emphasis on care coordination, the relationships between health professionals and healthcare organizations also must undergo major transformation. Specifically, greater alignment and integration of professionals and organizations is required to respond to these changes and to ensure the viability of both groups. However, unlike past organizational arrangements designed to align professional and organizational goals based on the dominance of either organizational or professional interests, we argue that arrangements characterized by multiple power centers and mutual influence are likely to have the greatest chance of success. These conjoint arrangements will not assume a single form but instead vary from highly structured single organizations that incorporate professionals as employees to networks of organizations and professional groups connected by contracts and common information systems. Regardless of the specific form taken, mechanisms to accommodate both macro care issues related to maximizing outcomes for populations of patients and micro care issues related to the care and preferences of individual patients will represent the defining features of these new organizations.

References

Agency for Healthcare Research and Quality. (May 8, 2014). *The state of Accountable Care Organizations*. Retrieved from https://innovations.ahrq.gov/perspectives/state-accountable-care-organizations

Alexander, J. A., Morlock, L. L., & Gifford, D. D. (1988). The effects of corporate restructuring on hospital policymaking. *Health Services Research, 23*(2), 311–337.

Alexander, J. A., Waters, T., Henderson, S., Burns, L, Shortell, S., Budetti, P. . . . Zuckerman, H. (2001). Risk assumption and physician alignment with health care systems. *Medical Care, 39*(7), 46–61.

Alexander, J. A., & Young, G. J., Weiner, B.J. & Hearld, L. R. (2009). How do system-affiliated hospitals fare in providing community benefit? *Inquiry, 46*(1), 72–90.

Alexander, J. A., & Young, G. J. (2010). Overcoming barriers to improved hospital-physician collaboration and alignment: Governance issues. In J. Crossan & L. Tollen (Eds.) *Partners in health: how physicians and hospitals can be accountable together* (pp. 141–168). San Francisco, CA: Jossey Bass.

Aucott, J. N., Pelecanos, E., Bailey, A. J., Shupe, T. C., Romeo, J. H., Ravdin, J. I., & Aron, D. C. (1995). Interdisciplinary integration for quality improvement: The Cleveland Veterans Affairs Medical Center firm system. *Joint Commission Journal Quality Improvement, 21,* 179–190.

Bazzoli, G. (2004). The corporatization of American hospitals. *Journal of Health Politics, Policy and Law, 29*(4-5), 885–905.

Beisecker, A. E., & Beisecker, T. D. (1993). Using metaphors to characterize doctor-patient relationships: Paternalism versus consumerism. *Health Communication, 5*(1), 41–58.

Boev, C., & Xia, Y. (2015). Nurse-physician collaboration and hospital-acquired infections in critical care. *Critical Care Nurse, 35*(2), 66–72.

Brody, D. (1980). The patient's role in clinical decision-making. *Annals of Internal Medicine, 93*(5), 718–722.

Burns, L. R., Andersen, R. M., & Shortell, R. M. (1990). The effect of hospital control strategies on physician satisfaction and hospital–physician conflict. *Health Services Research, 25,* 527–560.

Burns, L. R., Shortell, S. M., & Andersen, R. M. (1998). Does familiarity breed contentment? Attitudes and behaviors of integrated physicians. In J. Kronenfeld, (Ed.) *Research in the sociology of health care* (pp. 85–110). Greenwich, CT: JAI Press.

Butcher, L. (2008). Many changes in store as physicians become employees. *Managed Care.* Retrieved from http://www.managedcaremag.com/archives/0807/0807.physicians.html

Casalino, L. P., Wu, F. M., Ryan, A.M., Copeland, K., Rittenhouse, D. R., Ramsay, P. P., & Shortell, S. M. (2013). Independent practice associations and physician-hospital organizations can improve care management for smaller practices. *Health Affairs, 32*(8), 1376–1382.

Cassidy, A. (October 25, 2012). Nurse practitioners and primary care. *Health Affairs.* Retrieved from http://healthaffairs.org/healthpolicybriefs/brief_pdfs/healthpolicybrief_79.pdf

Charles, C., Whelan, T., & Gafni, A. (1999). What do we mean by partnership in making decisions about treatment? *British Medical Journal, 319*(7212), 780–782.

Charns, M. P., & Tewksbury, L. J. S. (1993). *Collaborative management in health care. Implementing the integrative organization.* San Francisco, CA: Jossey-Bass.

Dowell, M. (December 10, 2010). Co-management re-emerges as hospital-physician integration option. *Hospital Association of Southern California.* Retrieved from http://www.hasc.org/briefs-focus/co-management-re-emerges-hospital-physician-integration-option

Dukerich, J. M., Golden, B. R., & Shortell, S. M. (2002). Beauty is in the eye of the beholder: The impact of organizational identification, identity, and image on the cooperative behaviors of physicians. *Administrative Science Quarterly, 47,* 507–533.

Dupree, J. M., Patel, K., Singer, S., West, M., Wang, R., Zinner, M., & Weissman, J. (2014). Attention to surgeons and surgical care is largely missing from early Medicare Accountable Care Organizations, *Health Affairs, 33*(6), 972–979.

Everett, C. M., Thorpe, C. T., Palta, M. Carayon, P. Gilchrist, V. J., & Smith, M. A. (2013). Division of primary care services between physicians, physician assistants, and nurse practitioners to older patients with diabetes. *Medical Care Research and Review, 70*(5), 531–541.

Federal Trade Commission. (March 2014). *Competition and the regulation of advanced nurse practitioners.* Retrieved from https://www.ftc.gov/system/files/documents/reports/policy-perspectives-competition-regulation-advanced-practice-nurses/140307aprnpolicypaper.pdf

Fisher, E. S., Staiger, D. O., Bynum, J., & Gottlieb, D. J. (2006). Creating accountable care organizations: The extended hospital medical staff. *Health Affairs, 26*(1), w44–w57.

Freidson, E. (1970). *Professional dominance: The social structure of medical care.* Chicago, IL: Aldine Publishing Company.

Freidson, E. (1984). The changing nature of professional control. *American Review of Sociology, 10*, 1–20.

Gardner, D. (2010). Expanding scope of practice: Inter-professional collaboration or conflict. *Nursing Economics, 28*(4), 264–266.

Garman, A. N., Leach, D. C., & Spector, N. (2006). Worldviews in collision: Conflict and collaboration across professional lines. *Journal of Organizational Behavior, 27*(7), 829–849.

Gbemudu, J. N., Larson, B. K., VanCitters, A. D., Kreindler, S. A. Wu, F. M., Nelson, E. C., . . . Fisher, E. S. (January 2012). Healthcare partners: Building on a foundation of global risk management to achieve accountable care. *The Commonwealth Fund.* Retrieved from http://www.commonwealthfund.org/publications/case-studies/2012/jan/healthcare-partners

Grumbach, K., & Bodenheimer, T. (2004). Can health care teams improve primary care practice? *Journal of the American Medical Association, 291*(10), 1246–1251.

Guterman, S., Davis, K., Stremikis, K., & Drake, H. (2010). Innovation in Medicare and Medicaid will be central to health reform's success. *Health Affairs, 29*(6), 1188–1193.

Hain, D., & Fleck, L. M. (May 31, 2014). Barriers to NP practices that impact healthcare redesign. *The Online Journal of Issues in Nursing, 19*(2). Retrieved from http://www.nursingworld.org/MainMenuCategories/ANAMarketplace/ANAPeriodicals/OJIN/TableofContents/Vol-19-2014/No2-May-2014/Barriers-to-NP-Practice.html

Hastings, S. E., Armitrage, G. D., Mallinson, S., Jackson, K., & Suter, E. (2014). Exploring the systematic relationship between governance mechanisms in healthcare and health workforce outcomes: A systematic review. *BMC Health Services Research, 14*, 479.

Hekman, D. R., Bigley, G. A., Steensma, H. K., & Hereford, J. F. (2009). Combined effects of organizational and professional identification on the reciprocity dynamic for professional employees. *Academy of Management Journal, 52*(3), 506–526.

Hosler, F. W., & Nadle, P. A. (2000). Physician-hospital partnerships: Incentive alignment through shared governance within a performance improvement structure. *Joint Commission Journal on Quality Improvement, 26*, 59–73.

Institute of Medicine (IOM). (2000). *To err is human: Building a safer health system.* L. T. Kohn, J. M. Corrigan, & M. S. Donaldson (Eds.). Washington, DC: National Academies Press.

IOM. (2001). *Crossing the quality chasm: A new health system for the 21st century.* Washington, DC: National Academies Press.

IOM. (2003). Proceedings from Committee on the Health Professions Education Summit: *Health professions education: A bridge to quality.* A. C. Greiner & E. Knebel (Eds.). Washington, DC: National Academies Press.

IOM and National Academy of Engineering (2011). Engineering a Learning Healthcare System. Washington DC: National Academies Press.

Jurgeleit, P. B. (1997). Physician employment under managed care: Toward a retaliatory discharge cause of action for HMO-affiliated physicians. *Indiana Law Journal, 5*(1), 255–296.

Kitchener, M., Caronna, C. A., & Shortell, S. M. (2005). From the doctor's workshop to the iron cage? Evolving modes of physician contrail in US health systems. *Social Science & Medicine, 60*, 1131–1132.

Kocher, R., & Sahni, N. R. (2011). Hospitals' race to employ physicians—The logic behind a money-losing proposition. *New England Journal of Medicine, 364*(19), 1790–1793.

Kralewski, J., Rich, E., Feldman, R., Dowd, B., Bernhardt, T., Johnson, C., & Gold, W. (2000). Effects of medical group practice and physician payment methods on cost of care. *Health Services Research, 35*(3), 591–613.

Leape, L. L, & Berwick, D. M. (2005). Five years after To Err Is Human: What have we learned? *Journal of the American Medical Association, 293*(19), 2384–2390.

Lemieux-Charles, L., & McGuire, W. L. (2006). What do we know about health care team effectiveness? A review of the literature. *Medical Care Research and Review, 63*(3), 263–300.

Levay, C. & Waks, C. (2009). Professions and the pursuit of transparency in healthcare: Two cases of soft autonomy. *Organizational Studies, 30*(5), 509–527.

Levick, D. (September 25, 1995). Cigna to sell assets of its biggest HMO. *Hartford Courant*. Retrieved from http://articles.courant.com/1995-09-29/business/9509290017_1_cigna-healthcare-cigna-medical-group-cigna-deal

Lichtenstein, R., Alexander, J. A., Wells, R., & McCarthy, J. (2004). Status differences in cross-functional teams: Effects on individual member participation, job satisfaction, and intent to quit. *Journal of Health and Social Behavior, 45*(3), 322–335.

Lindeke, L. L., & Sieckert, A. S. (January 31, 2005). Nurse-physician workplace collaboration. *The Online Journal of Issues in Nursing, 10*(1), Manuscript 4.

McConnel, K. J., Lindrooth, R. C., Wholey, D. R., & Bloom, N. (2013). Management practices and the quality of care in cardiac units. *Journal of the American Medical Association Internal Medicine, 173*(8), 648–692.

Mitchell, P. M., Wynia, R., Golden, B., McNellis, S., Okun, C. E., Webb, V., . . . Von Kohorn, I. (2012). *Core principles & values of effective team-based health care.* Discussion Paper, Washington, DC: Institute of Medicine.

Morrisey, M. A., Alexander, J. A., Burns, L. R., & Johnson, V. (1996). Managed care and physician/hospital integration. *Health Affairs, 15*, 62.

Nelson, E. C., Batalden, P. B., Huber, T. P., Mohr, J. J., Godfrey, M. M. Headrick, L. A., & Wasson, J. H. (2002). Microsystems in health care: Part 1. Learning from high-performing front-line clinical units. *Joint Commission Journal on Quality Improvement 28*, 472–497.

Nembhard, I. M., Alexander, J. A, Hoff, T., & Ramanujam, R. (2009). Why does the quality of health care continue to lag? Insights from management research. *Academy of Management Perspectives, 23*(1), 1–27.

O'Daniel, M., & Rosenstein, A. H. (2008). Professional communication and team collaboration, in patient safety and quality: An evidence-based handbook for nurses. R. G. Hughes (Ed.). Rockville, MD: Agency for Healthcare Research and Quality.

Parker, V., Charns, M., & Young, G. (2001). Clinical service lines: An initial framework and empirical exploration. *Journal of Healthcare Management, 46*, 261–276.

Pauly, M., & Redisch, M. (1973). The non-for-profit hospital as a physicians' cooperative. *The American Economic Review, 63*(1), 87–99.

Rundall, T., Alexander, J. A., & Shortell, S. (2005). Contending institutional logics: An organizational-economic theory of physician-hospital integration, resistance and change. *Journal of Health and Social Behavior, 46*(1), 121–135.

Scott, W. R. (1982). Managing professional work: Three models of control for health organizations. *Health Services Research, 17*, 213–240.

Scott, W. R., & Davis, G. F. (2007). *Organizations and organizing: Rational, natural and open system perspectives.* New York, NY: Pearson Education.

Shields, M. C., Patel, P. H., Manning, M., & Sacks, L. (2011). A model for integrating independent physicians into accountable care organizations. *Health Affairs, 30*(1), 161–172.

Smith, M., Bates, D. W., & Bodenheimer, T. S. (2013). Pharmacists belong in accountable care organizations and integrated care teams. *Health Affairs, 32*(11), 1963–1970.

Starr, P. M. (1982). *The social transformation of American medicine.* New York, NY: Basic Books.

Sullivan, K. (August 4, 2014). Three strategies to promote a hospital culture of ownership. *FierceHealthcare.* Retrieved from http://www.fiercehealthcare.com/story/3-strategies-promote-hospital-culture-ownership/2014-08-04

Taylor, N., Clay-Williams, R., Hogden, E., Braithwaite, J., & Groene, O. (2015). High performing hospitals: A qualitative systematic review of associated factors and practical strategies for improvement. *BMC Health Services Research, 15*(244), 2–22.

Truog, R. D. (2012). Patients and doctors: The evolution of a relationship. *New England Journal of Medicine, 266*(7), 581–585.

Tye, J. (December 12, 2012). Building a culture of ownership in health care. *Hospital and Health Networks.* Retrieved from http://www.hhnmag.com/Daily/2012/Dec/tye121212-1540003951

Van Der Vegt, G. S., & Bunderson, J. S. (2005). Learning and performance in multidisciplinary teams: The importance of collective team identification, *Academy of Management Journal, 48*(3), 377–386.

Viggiano, T. R., Pawlina, W., Lindor, K. D., Olsen, K. D., & Cortese, D. A. (2007). Putting the needs of the patient first: Mayo clinic's core value, institutional culture, and professionalism covenant. *Academic Medicine, 82*(11), 1089–1093.

Weinberg, D. B. (2003). *Code green: Money-driven hospitals and the dismantling of nursing.* Ithaca, NY: ILR Press/Cornell University Press.

Young, G. J., Beckman, H., Baker, E. (2012). Financial incentives, professional values and performance: A study of pay-for-performance in a professional organization. *Journal of Organizational Behavior, 33,* 964–983.

Young, G. J., Charns, M., & Hereen, T. (2004). Product line management in professional organizations: An empirical test of competing theoretical perspectives. *Academy of Management Journal, 47,* 723–734.

Young, G. J., Desai, K., & Hellinger, F. (2000). Community control and the pricing patterns of nonprofit hospitals: an antitrust analysis. *Journal of Health Politics, Policy and Law, 25,* 1051–1082.

Young, D. W., & Saltman, R. B. (1985). *The Hospital Power Equilibrium.* Baltimore, MD: The Johns Hopkins University Press.

COMMENTARY TO ACCOMPANY CHAPTER 4

Lynne Eickholt

THIS CHAPTER OPENS with a very brief summary of the cultural norms in the healthcare professions, particularly among physicians, that have reinforced professional autonomy and stymied integration of professionals in hospital and health system operations in ways that promote greater efficiency and better quality. The chapter continues with a brief summary of the healthcare reform forces applying pressure to healthcare organizations and their allied medical professions into new models that will support the integration and alignment necessary for long term success.

How to align physicians with hospitals and health systems in pursuit of goals that respond to the new value-based purchasing requirements of the federal government, state governments, insurers, and employers is a central issue for all healthcare organizations. All health system forums that this commentator attends have frequent discussion sessions and programs focused on "physician–health system alignment." One forum of the 100 largest health systems in the country published the findings from interviews with executives at 26 systems on the challenges of health system–physician alignment, and at the request of its members, it recently conducted a survey of the governance structures for employed medical groups.

I would underscore this chapter's summary of the massive changes in healthcare that are at odds with the traditional culture of the medical professions and are driving the need for professional and health system alignment. First, the practice of medicine has become so complex that physicians cannot possibly maintain all the knowledge in their own heads. My organization has been a leader in developing clinical decision support systems and is spending a substantial sum to install a sophisticated electronic medical record system that contains such support to aid clinicians in care decisions. The development of such a system cannot be funded, developed, or effectively deployed by autonomous physicians operating in their subspecialty domains. To paraphrase a physician colleague of mine, "a great physician with no supporting infrastructure will be merely average, and an average physician with great infrastructure will be good."

In addition to the evolution of medical care requiring new models of professional and administrative alignment, breath taking changes in public policy regarding the funding and delivery of healthcare require rapid reorganization of the healthcare delivery system. Through the Affordable Care Act and subsequent regulatory changes, the Centers for Medicare & Medicaid Services (CMS) is paying healthcare organizations and physicians for achieving quality and efficiency targets. Also, the CMS is promoting risk-based payments to healthcare organizations that must work with their allied physicians across specialties to achieve both quality and cost targets for either defined health episodes, such as 90 days of care for hip and knee replacements, or all care for an enrolled population. The private insurance sector is rapidly following suit. Healthcare organizations without effective physician alignment strategies will not prosper.

The authors identify an opposite pole from the autonomy tradition—what they term heteronomous relationships, where physicians fall under the larger authority of the health system or hospital—and note that research shows little success in this approach. The authors suggest a middle ground of conjoint physician administrative structures that has five important elements—joint governance structures, robust information on practices and care delivery, team-based care, aligned incentives, and a "culture of ownership" among healthcare providers.

In my experience with my own delivery system and those of my colleagues in strategy, we all are trying to find the right conjoint structure. In addition to the long-standing academic practice organizations closely integrated with the two academic hospitals, my organization is working to develop a robust and influential community physician organization that unites both employed and affiliated physicians in pursuit of common goals. In the survey mentioned earlier of large integrated delivery systems, executives identified challenges in physician alignment that reflect most of the five elements identified as important to effective conjoint structures—integration as full senior partner of the system on par with the hospitals, conversion of separate medical records to an enterprise system, the right incentives to transition from fee-for-service to value-based care, and moving from a physician group culture to one of "systemness."

As the authors note, the area of physician–health system relationships is ripe for research. Given the wealth of information now publicly available on quality and patient satisfaction, in addition to financial and market results, it is possible to test how different forms of conjoint governance result in organizational success. One such study of academic medical center integration between faculty practices and hospital–health systems done by the consulting group ECG Management Consultants recently came across my desk. Academic medical centers were rated as more or less integrated based on structural as well as functional characteristics, including collaborative strategic planning, budgeting, capital, facilities and clinical service planning, physician recruitment, and matrix reporting. The study found that more integrated academic health systems performed better on reputation, quality, research funds awarded, and strength of training programs, but not in terms of finances. More work on how to objectively measure and quantify the degree of functional integration between health systems and medical professionals would enable similar highly valuable research into comparative effectiveness of different organizational structures and provide an evidence base for healthcare executives struggling to manage this critical element of organizational change and success.

5

THE PARADOXES OF LEADING AND MANAGING

HEALTHCARE PROFESSIONALS

Toward the Integration of Healthcare Services

Mirko Noordegraaf and Lawton Robert Burns

Introduction

Eliot Freidson (2001) described professionalism as an alternative model for organizing and controlling work distinct from bureaucracy and the free market
of economic exchange. According to Freidson, professionalism contains five elements: (1) a body of specialized knowledge and skill that requires the exercise of
considerable discretion; (2) the division of labor based on functional specialization, with assistant roles controlled by the occupation; (3) restricted professional
entry based on stipulated training, also controlled by the occupation; (4) training
programs that produce the credentialed practitioners, also controlled by the occupation; and (5) an ideology that serves transcendent values and places primacy on
social benefits over economic rewards. Beyond Freidson's ideal type, research on
professionalism has emphasized an occupational culture based on a set of values
(e.g., code of ethics) and commitments (e.g., to excellence, quality, public service,
and client welfare), often developed through socialization during training, as well
as through occupational identification with one's colleagues and professional associations (Wynd, 2003; Brint, 2006). Freidson's model describes the reality of one
group of healthcare professionals (physicians) and the aspirations of most others
(nurses, pharmacists, social workers). Physicians in the United States have enjoyed
a monopoly over most of the major decisions that drive the cost and utilization of

healthcare services: hospital admission, hospital discharge, specialist referral (in tightly managed care settings), prescription of a medication, performance of surgery, and conduct of diagnostic testing. In controlling these activities, physicians account for roughly 85% of all healthcare spending—either directly through their own activities, or indirectly through the work of other professionals and institutions ordered by physicians to help treat their patients (Eisenberg, 2002; Sager & Socolar, 2005). Nonphysician professions seek greater responsibility, autonomy, and control over the content of their work—embodied in the phrase "practice at the top of their license." In the past, their work has more typically been directly overseen by physicians or at least based on physician orders. At present, some professional groups, such as nurse anesthetists, midwives, advance practice nurses, and nurse practitioners, seek greater authority from state governments to practice with less physician supervision.

The professional elements and orientations described above are embodied in the diverse roles that professionals play. Physicians and nurses both occupy multiple roles; most of them are profession-centric. Physician roles include patient's agent, self-interested economic agent, and society's agent (Eisenberg, 1986). Professional nurse roles include client advocate, change agent, caregiver, teacher, counselor, and coordinator (of lower-level personnel). Only one of nursing's roles is that of "colleague" (Hood, 2014).

Tellingly, some of these nonphysician medical professionals espouse values very similar to those of physicians. For example, a major text on professional nursing cites the values of caring, compassion, commitment, competence, and confidence (Hood, 2014). Moreover, each of the various healthcare professions has its own professional associations, professional journals, training institutions, credentialing systems, and practice models and organizations. None of them explicitly includes "collaboration" or "teamwork" with the others as part of its professional identity (see Buerki & Vottero, 2002; Wynd, 2003). Thus, they constitute silos of knowledge and knowledge workers in the healthcare system. This is a major contributor to the *fragmentation* so often used to describe the system. The problem of professional fragmentation is compounded by fragmentation in the delivery sites (e.g., many small physician offices, many hospitals), the increasing specialization of the medical and nursing workforces, and other divisive forces that fragment healthcare professionals (e.g., Elhauge, 2010; Hoff, 2013).

Such fragmentation or differentiation unavoidably calls for corresponding *integration* (Lawrence & Lorsch, 1967). Industry analysts have long championed integrative and collaborative mechanisms to counteract the centrifugal tendencies fostered by professional silos, functional specialization, and organizational fragmentation (Lehman, 1975; Charns & Tewskbury, 1993). Such calls have received new emphasis in recent efforts to promote patient-centered medical homes (PCMHs), care coordination programs, clinical microsystems of care, integrated delivery networks (IDNs), and accountable care organizations (ACOs). Such integrative and collaborative mechanisms are largely organizational in nature. As such, they require new leadership and managerial skills on the part of the professional groups whose work is to be coordinated. In sum, there are growing pressures today to counterbalance the specialized and autonomous work of healthcare professionals with the need for collaborative models that integrate their work efforts in organized settings of care.

But such collaborative models face incredible headwinds. There is a lack of an evidence base for the ability of several of these models to reduce cost and improve quality of care. Moreover, surveys reveal that clinicians express mixed views about the ability of such structures to improve the quality of care they render to patients (Ryan et al., 2015). Physicians are less sanguine about their prospects than nurse practitioners and physician assistants. Such divergent opinions may make professional collaboration and thus organizational success more difficult to achieve. Additional evidence suggests that *collaborative capacity* may be more important than "collaborative structures" to foster interdependence, quality interactions, and collaborative influence among team members. Collaborative capacity is defined here as the routines and work processes— often embedded in work cultures, decision-making styles, shared commitments, and team dynamics—that foster coordinated behavior among professionals and other stakeholders. Such capacity is promoted by patient-centered values and supportive contexts but constrained by the division of labor and status hierarchy among the healthcare professions (Weinberg, Cooney-Miner, Perloff, Babington, & Avgar, 2011). Our understanding of collaborative capacity is constrained by the focus of most research on the *structures* rather than the *processes* of collaboration (Song, Ryan, Tendulkar et al., 2015; Valentijn, Ruwaard, Vrijhoef et al., 2015). This chapter reviews what care providers can do to stimulate collaborative capacity and recent efforts to develop collaborative routines and processes. We explore leadership and management implications and discuss how integrated care can be established by connecting healthcare institutions, workforces, and values.

The Paradox of Professionalism and Collaboration

The traditional model of professional work and professionalism runs counter to the current imperative for professionals to collaborate and work in teams. An Institute of Medicine (2011) report identifies nurse–physician collaboration as one of its top four priorities to help redesign healthcare in the United States. A recent research study suggests that such collaboration helps reduce hospital-acquired infections (Boev & Xia, 2015). The changing healthcare context of consumerism, standardization, shared governance, and accountability (for both quality and cost) requires healthcare professionals to engage in more collaborative action in healthcare delivery. But this context also creates a paradoxical situation for healthcare workers.

On the one hand, professionals need to develop new organizational and occupational approaches to ensure high-quality care such as:

- Multidisciplinary teams and treatment
- Integrated care teams and microsystems of care
- Visible checklists that regulate patient care
- Client-based innovation that relies on technologies for keeping track of patient flows and interacting with patients
- Healthcare networks that link medical interventions inside and outside hospitals that cross the care continuum

New work models entail closer monitoring of professional activity and provision of feedback to professionals on their activity. Notifications of possible deviations from practice norms of their colleagues and practice guidelines issued by professional societies, reduce variations in their work with an aim to improve its quality and to streamline clinical processes.

On the other hand, these very same changes make collaborative action challenging, at least for physicians. Consumerism, externally developed quality standards, and practice model innovations represent external pressures on medical practice, which has not changed much in the past decades. Moreover, embracing such changes has never been part of the bedrock of medical professionalism. These also threaten the medical profession's traditional boundaries with patients (who traditionally just played "the sick role"), nonphysician professions (who took their orders from or received orders for their services from physicians), hospitals (which served as the physician's workshop), and payers (who traditionally were outside third parties that just paid the bills incurred).

The paradox can be restated in more familiar terms. Professionalism rests on a bedrock of specialized knowledge and an organization of similarly trained specialists around one another. Such focus, specialization, and colocation confer scale economies and productivity in human resources, training, and professional learning. On the other hand, collaboration rests on a bedrock of diversified inputs, reduced transaction costs among the specialized players, and on improved coordination among them. The paradox is thus somewhat akin to the tradeoffs in switching from the invisible hand of the market to the visible hand of the corporate hierarchy (Chandler, 1977).

Not surprisingly, calls for collaborative work design pose difficulties for physicians, who are used to being "captain of the ship." Already, more than 40% of physicians surveyed report they are burned out and/or dissatisfied with their jobs (Shanafelt et al., 2012; Jauhar, 2014; Jackson Healthcare, 2015). At the same time physicians are being asked to change their workflows and care relationships, they are experiencing stagnant incomes, declining status, diminished respect from patients, greater pressures to be more productive (i.e., see more patients), more paperwork from payers, increased pressure from a rise in their chronic care caseload, and increasing blame for cost and quality issues.

Ironically, changes to new work models may also pose difficulties for nonphysician professions (e.g., nursing) that have undertaken their own professionalizing efforts and sought greater autonomy from physicians for decades. The nonphysician professions have their own distinctive work cultures that include values, guidelines, routines, and codes of conduct that deviate not only from physicians but other professional groups. Moreover, these professions may themselves be stratified, whereby some professions (e.g., nurses) might actually be (or at least see themselves as) more valued and superior to the others and thus more likely to exercise decision-making control over the others. Such professional boundaries thus extend beyond just physicians. They can affect day-to-day interactions among different professional groups as well as their attempts to adapt to new ways of working together.

Nevertheless, the practice model changes are likely less threatening to nurses and other nonphysician professionals, given their historically subordinate role in patient decision-making. New collaborative models may therefore be more welcomed by the nonphysician medical professions because these models give more recognition to the nonphysicians as important team members, afford them more voice in decision-making, and reduce the status differentials among them. For all of these reasons, however, the new models are likely to be resisted most by physicians.

Indeed, it is possible that these changes may lead to so-called jurisdictional battles between the healthcare professions (see Abbott, 1988). This especially happens when one profession is forced to adjust its actions in light of the actions of another, when existing professions assume new tasks and/or identities (e.g., nurses who become nurse physicians), and when new professions emerge (e.g., care coordinators). This is not only a matter of privilege, power, and prestige, but also of conflicting expertise and identities. Different professions have distinctive *ways of knowing*, which are reflected in ideas, expert and often tacit knowledge, and evidence. They have distinctive *ways of being*, which are reflected in their values, professional identities, and reference groups. And they have distinctive *ways of acting*, which include specific methods, techniques, ways of working, and routines. These elements of professional work are difficult to align, especially given the lack of definitive proof for deciding which ideas and acts are "the best," and the complexity of work situations and the "trial-and-error" nature of many work processes.

All of this fragments professional domains and makes professional action more interdependent as well as more dependent on nonprofessional actors (e.g., hospitals, payers, regulators). Professional domains will not passively adjust, but instead either actively resist adaptations or proactively seek new ways to provide healthcare that fit their ideas and own separate identities and interests. Such centrifugal forces need to be counterbalanced by centripetal forces that promote *collaboration* and *integrated care* by teams of professionals, aimed at connecting instead of separating different ideas, identities, and interests. These centralizing forces are difficult to exercise in virtual settings, including loosely linked referral networks of physicians, continua of care involving home health agencies, physicians, and hospitals, as well as independent practice associations (IPAs) (Mehrotra, Epstein, & Rosenthal, 2006; Burns, Goldsmith, & Sen, 2013). This fragmentation is accentuated by the geographic separation of different professionals and the reliance on information technology (e.g., electronic medical records) as opposed to face-to-face interactions to coordinate their efforts.

In contrast, these centralizing activities may be more easily practiced in organized settings of healthcare delivery where members of the different professional groups are at least colocated and can assemble together around the patient. However, colocation is insufficient to guarantee the needed collaboration. Physicians, nurses, pharmacists, and other professionals engaged in patient care need to exercise leadership and coordination to break down the boundaries that separate them, to develop collaborative models and joint decision-making with other professionals, and encourage their colleagues to participate. Both the leaders of these efforts as well as the rank-and-file participants also require training and education to improve the working of these collaborative models. In this manner, the push for collaboration places a premium on leadership and management: *leadership* in order to adapt healthcare institutions and their values to contemporary requirements and *management* to coordinate workers and workforces in healthcare. Later on, we explore these leadership and management consequences and discuss the rise of more *integrated* care accompanied by collaborative capacity. But first, we elaborate calls for collaboration and the obstacles and divisive forces that have to be overcome.

Calls for (and Obstacles to) Collaboration

Changing contexts that alter the conditions for healthcare delivery have been extensively discussed earlier, and they are summarized in Chapter 1. We focus on one of the major consequences: healthcare professionals are expected to work together to deliver quality care. Team-based settings such as the Mayo Clinic, Cleveland Clinic, and CareMore are commonly preferred and recommended as models of excellent care—even by the President of the United States (Naymik, 2009). The various changes described in preceding chapters have reenergized the search for coordinated and integrated care (Crosson, 2009; Ham, Imison, Goodwin, Dixon, & South, 2011; Vize, 2012). In this new perspective, healthcare has become the product of collaborative efforts of professionals using:

- Well-organized procedures, such as care pathways, guidelines, and checklists
- Well-designed organizational systems, such as patient institutes and microsystems of care, based on well-functioning processes (teamwork, transitions)

All of these efforts are supposed to support the "triple aim." Here, physicians, nurses, pharmacists, and other healthcare professionals work together to render high-quality services at low cost to improve the patient experience (Berwick, Nolan, & Whittington, 2008).

At first sight, this search has been occasioned by new organizational and payment requirements. Providers are now asked to be accountable for both the quality and cost of care they render (e.g., pay-for-performance), and are increasingly paid on the basis of "value" (e.g., quality divided by cost). They must increasingly view their work as production processes that need to be streamlined using the techniques of lean manufacturing (e.g., Toyota Production System [TPS]). Streamlined work processes not only reduce expensive waste but also facilitate patient flow and patient convenience. Such managerial systems serve to optimize production and improve customer satisfaction. Patients must be served as smoothly as possible, based on their needs and desires, and with maximum customer orientation. Working together, streamlining healthcare processes and communicating well with other professionals and patients have all been recommended as new standards of modern professional work.

The push for demonstrated value fuels a long-running but slow-moving trend to force some healthcare professionals such as physicians to look beyond their traditional roles as patient agents and self-interested economic agents to embrace the additional role as society's and (given the trend in coordinated care and physician employment) the organization's agent (Eisenberg, 1986). Moses et al. (2013) describe these divergent roles as healthcare's "triangle of conflicting expectations." The same push for value also requires multiple professions to now submit to common governance models in which no one group is ascendant. The quintessential common governance model today is the ACO, in which all professions and specialties within a given profession must collaborate on seeking cost-effective care delivery in order to receive performance rewards. Advocates of collaboration recommend a "level playing field" among the various healthcare professionals (Robert Wood Johnson Foundation, 2015).

The push for integration is not solely or primarily due to organizational imperatives and reimbursement changes. Many societal transitions fuel the installment of new organizational systems and the need for collaboration (e.g., Adler, Kwon, & Heckscher, 2008; Noordegraaf, 2011, 2015; Adler & Kwon, 2013). Changing *patient health status*, for example, presents new challenges for healthcare provision. The spread of chronic disease and the growing prevalence of patients with comorbid conditions and multiple chronic illnesses involve more caregivers and services (both medical and social). This, in turn, requires the coordinated action of multiple professionals and thus multidisciplinary treatment by a range of physicians and nurse practitioners (e.g., Plochg, Klazinga, & Starfield, 2009). It also requires more sustained face-to-face interaction among diverse providers, more face-to-face interaction among providers and their patients and families, and an increased emphasis on wellness and prevention. The expanding and increasingly diverse array of needed services must rest on leadership and managerial supports to professional collaboration.

A second societal transition underway calls for healthcare professionals to embrace *disruptive innovations*, both organizational as well as technological, that promise more timely and convenient care (Burns, David, & Helmchen, 2011). Disruption is usually threatening to professionals. Professionals often resist "disruption" from within their own ranks in the form of paradigm shifts in training (e.g., team-based training in medical school) or treatment/therapy (e.g., port-access heart surgery); disruption from outside their ranks (e.g., nurse anesthetists, retail clinics, patient centered medical homes) is even more threatening to physicians. Disruptive innovations now in vogue, such as PCMHs, ACOs, and coordinated care organizations, commonly require professionals to work with (a) different professionals, (b) in new modes of reciprocal interaction, (c) in ways that reduce their status differentials, (d) in ways that cede more decision-making to other professionals, and (e) in ways that require electronic bases of collaboration (Peikes, Chen, Schore & Brown, 2009; Brown, 2013). The advent of "virtual supervision" (in which general practitioners electronically oversee the work of nurse practitioners in retail clinics) and "speedy diagnostics" (in which groups such as oncologists and radiologists work closely together, for example, to diagnose cancer as quickly as possible) fits societal calls for more efficient and better care.

A third societal transition calls for the reduction of *medical errors* and increased attention to *patient safety* (Vogus, Sutcliffe, & Weick, 2010; Sutcliffe, 2011). Patients and public alike focus on medical errors due to fears of suboptimal care *and* expectations of optimal care—faultless, low cost, and value adding. Although hospitals might respond by installing safety systems, guaranteeing safety has a lot to do with the actions of and interactions among healthcare professionals. Mistakes frequently occur during patient transitions, provider shift transitions (e.g., handovers), communication between caregivers, briefings, and joint decisions.

Boundaries imply that there are status and political differences between professionals. In the absence of conditions to establish "psychological safety," the "weaker" professional groups may be reluctant to speak up about problems in healthcare processes. To optimize preoperative, perioperative, and postoperative processes, healthcare organizations may utilize checklists, briefings, and time outs. However, such briefings and time outs are difficult to use amid dynamic and time-sensitive work processes. It is also sometimes difficult for nonphysician professions to actually stop the treatments conducted by physicians when things go wrong. According to Leistikow, Kalkman, and de Bruijn (2011), this explains "why patient safety is such a hard nut to crack." There are four key challenges in "implementing patient safety interventions:" visibility, ambiguity, complexity, and autonomy. Safety problems are often difficult to "see," both for patients as well as professionals. They are ambiguous, in that clear evidence on cause-and-effect relations is often inconclusive. They are complex due to the fact that many variables in a hospital context affect safety outcomes, varying from clean tiles to well-educated workers. Finally, professional autonomy makes it difficult for medical professionals to jointly tackle safety issues.

A fourth transition is the growing *ambulatory* and *outpatient care market,* and along with it the growing competition between hospitals and physicians to capture this market. There has been a marked shift from inpatient to outpatient care in the United States since 1980. Market growth rates and service profit margins are now much higher in the latter than the former. Hospitals, the traditional owner of the inpatient market, are now competing with members of their medical staffs, the traditional owner of the ambulatory market, for this business. Thus, at the same time that hospitals are trying to integrate with physicians and foster collaboration between physicians and other professionals, they are also now competing with them. Hospitals consequently have to figure out how to balance cooperation with competition. The situation has become more complicated for hospitals, because their medical staff members now spend less time seeing patients in the inpatient setting, affording hospitals less time to directly interact and have dialogues with their physicians.

Breaking Down Silos and Overcoming Divisive Forces

The challenge to achieve collaboration and integration is enormous. The societal transitions described above call for adaptations in professional practices and interprofessional interactions that encounter stiff headwinds. The (perceived) weakening of status, the loss of autonomy, and the pressures to adapt ways of working and routines all hinder the breaking down of professional silos. Boundaries are partly technical and functional, related to the usage of different methods, techniques, or terminologies. They are also moral and political, not in the least because they are established to protect values, convictions, and interests of distinctive professional segments that have learned to protect their fields and actions (e.g., Bucher & Strauss, 1961; Martin, Currie, & Finn, 2009).

US healthcare organizations are now actively seeking to alter (and hopefully improve) the quality and costs of the care they provide by reorganizing the work that their various professional groups perform. Such initiatives seek to overcome centrifugal forces, develop cross-boundary collaboration, and achieve integrated care. Some initiatives relate to new organizational structures, such as the creation of medical *professional service firms* to actively "manage care" (e.g., Scott, Ruef, Mendel, & Caronna, 2000; Empson, Muzio, Broschak, & Hinings, 2015). Some initiatives relate to the rise of *cooperation* in diversified systems (e.g., Hoff, 2013) to connect diverse groups working in organizational settings (see Noordegraaf, 2011, 2015), such as the use of *interactive steering* or *professional compacts*. Some initiatives stress the importance of *harmonious systems* (e.g., Mintzberg, 2012) in which gaps between higher levels of administration and lower levels of operation are reduced, thereby improving adaptability and decision-making.

The location and pursuit of these initiatives in organizational contexts is a necessary but insufficient condition for their success. To succeed, the organizations need to develop capabilities in professional leadership and management of these initiatives as well. Without professional steering and conduct, there is no professional acceptance. Without professional role modeling of the changes needed, there will be no template for other professionals to successfully emulate. The leadership activities undertaken include the following:

- New institutional structures that span professional groups
- New value-based contracts with their professional colleagues

- New organizational groupings that co-locate different professionals
- New processes that require them to conduct joint problem-solving

The new management activities undertaken include the following:

- Joint conduct of daily work
- Development of multidisciplinary teams
- Development of designated coordinators among professional workers
- Development of flexible models of integration that suit the preferences of individual professionals
- Development of new management tools, training, and education

The following sections highlight various ways to *lead* and *manage* healthcare professionals, which can serve to *integrate* professionals in organizational structures and processes that accommodate their professional ways of working. Leadership and managership have been distinguished in earlier research (Burns & Becker, 1987). Here we simply use the two terms to distinguish what (top) executives do to inspire, direct, and guide professionals and their institutions, and what (middle and lower) managerial levels do to coordinate workers and workforces in day-to-day healthcare delivery. In addition, we show how integrated care depends on sound *connections* between these institutions, workforces, and values.

Leading Healthcare Professionals and Their Institutions

Leadership involves several behaviors that are essential wherever the coordinated efforts of participants are desired (Burns, 1978). It involves establishing organizational values and institutionalizing them throughout the organizations (Selznick, 1957). Such institutional leadership entails moral efforts to embody these values and role model them for organizational participants (Burns & Becker, 1987). Leadership also entails symbolic efforts to ensure the organization's legitimacy (in the eyes of both internal and external stakeholders) and provide a sense of stability and self-control. Finally, leadership entails the use of proactive efforts (e.g., new strategic initiatives) that challenge organizational participants to envision and embrace new, valued models of organizing and work. Such efforts have been used to promote collaboration among healthcare professionals and between professionals and the bureaucracies in which they work. Below we highlight the use of organizational compacts, leadership dyads, microsystems and patient institutes, and other efforts to break down boundaries between professionals in healthcare organizations.

ORGANIZATIONAL COMPACTS

Some healthcare organizations have sought to redefine their relationships with key professional groups (e.g., physicians) and overcome the divide between administrative and professional cultures and forms of work. Such a divide leads to divergent views on appropriate strategies to pursue, can be organize work, allocate resources, way to make decisions, and the appropriate core values of the organization. There is no comparable literature on hospital–nurse compacts, perhaps reflecting the reality that the nursing organization is already part of the hospital's administrative hierarchy. By contrast, the medical organization is a separate, self-governing entity that functions outside the administrative hierarchy according to standards set by The Joint Commission.

One vehicle for bridging this divide is the "personal compact." Personal compacts have three dimensions: (1) a formal dimension that can contain job descriptions, employment contracts, performance agreements, and the authority and resources to do one's job; (2) a social dimension that includes management integrity (e.g., commitment to fulfill promises) and shared values to uphold; and (3) a psychological dimension that includes personal commitment and loyalty, trust, a sense of mutual dependence, and recognition along with other intrinsic rewards.

These compacts are basically new covenants that try to shift away from utilitarian exchange to more normative exchange. Utilitarianism underlies the traditional transactional exchanges between the voluntary medical staff and the hospital. Under the traditional model, physicians bring their patients to the hospital and feed the hospital's top-line revenue; in exchange, they are permitted to utilize the hospital and its staff as resources serving the "doctor's workshop" (Pauly & Redisch, 1973). Physician compacts seek to replace this utilitarian model with a more value-laden agreement that spells out the commitments of the organization to the physician and the commitments of the physician to the organization. Such commitments are as much normative as utilitarian—for example, emphasizing quality improvement, organizational citizenship, resource stewardship, and patient safety. They are also viewed as an initial step taken to prepare for stronger interprofessional collaboration in the future (Robert Wood Johnson Foundation, 2015).

This movement reflects the broader trend toward "psychological contracts," which set forth (in more explicit terms than in typical employment contracts) the mutual promises, expectations, and obligations of the employer and employee. They are thus more promissory and reciprocal than traditional contracts (Rousseau, 1990). One research field investigation examined the character of the personal compacts developed by a large hospital system (Allina Health System) with its new, employed large group of primary care physicians (Bunderson, Lofstrom, & Van de Ven, 1998).

These compacts were designed to support the system's effort to develop one of the nation's first IDNs including hospitals, physicians, and a health plan—similar to the Kaiser model. Despite the existence of these compacts, the paradox between professionalism and coordination persisted. The study found that the system's lay managers preferred a system oriented more to bureaucratic and market models that emphasized system goals and coordination, business orientation, and competition. By contrast, physicians were more oriented to professional and community models that emphasized clinical excellence and quality, professional control and identity, and community health and access issues.

A second study reported more favorable results from system efforts to replace the "implicit compact" with its physicians with a more "explicit compact" (Bohmer & Ferlins, 2008). The former compact emphasized physician autonomy, protection from the economic environment, and professional entitlement; the latter compact emphasized quality improvement, patient focus, collaboration, and embracing change. The new compact was developed to counter low physician morale in a large multispecialty group that had encountered its first operating loss in 100 years and was now subjected to cost-cutting measures. The new compact became embedded in physician performance reviews and a new incentive compensation system, both of which now included group as well as individual metrics. Metrics included in the group effort component included relationship with and respect for other members of the care team, embracing evidence-based practice, and participating in organizational change and improvement.

LEADERSHIP DYADS: PHYSICIAN AND EXECUTIVES

Some hospitals have sought to pair physicians and lay executives at top managerial levels to "role model" an important new attitude and behavior: (a) leadership commitment to interprofessional collaboration between the two hierarchies and (b) demonstration of the interpersonal relationships needed in action. Such dyads can be subsequently replicated at middle and lower levels of management as well. This trend has been characterized as the "Noah's Ark" of management (two by two), with physician–manager teams at the executive level, the clinical level, and the patient floor level. Such personnel dyads are designed to bring together the clinical and administrative hierarchies to provide voice to both perspectives, to allow joint decision-making, and to facilitate more effective matrix management. Such an approach was also used in the formation of the Allina Health System (Bunderson et al., 1998).

There is no empirical evidence whether such dyads are successful. However, there is anecdotal evidence that the dyadic approach is an important ingredient to the quality improvement efforts undertaken by some health systems (Robert Wood Johnson Foundation, 2015). Indeed, dyads have become a common solution to the problems faced by hospitals that seek to "integrate" or "align" with their medical staffs in the pursuit of IDN formation, accountable care, and population health. These dyads may be found at various levels in a hospital system and used to oversee an integrated clinical service line (e.g., cardiovascular, orthopedics, cancer care), divisions of care providers (e.g., regional primary care networks), or alternative delivery systems.

There is a natural division of labor in these dyads (Zismer, Brueggemann, & James, 2010). The physician manager has responsibility for quality of the clinical work, provider behavior, provider productivity, clinical innovation, compliance, patient care standards, clinical pathway management, and referring physician relations. By contrast, the lay manager has responsibility for operations, revenue management, operating expense management, capital planning and allocation, staffing, performance reporting, supply chain management, and support systems and services. The two managers and their hierarchies come together to jointly conduct a third set of activities: vision, values, strategy, culture, and overall performance.

LEADERSHIP DYADS: PHYSICIANS AND NURSES

In addition to physician–manager dyads, some healthcare organizations also place physician–nurse dyads in charge of clinical areas. These dyads are designed to promote teamwork between the two major professional groups responsible for patient care. They can also serve as a vehicle to train both sets of professionals in the business management of clinical areas—for example, by giving them responsibility for profit and loss, budgeting, and personnel—and thereby serve as a clinician leadership track.

These dyads are first demonstrated in the C-suite between the Chief Medical Officer (CMO) and Chief Nursing Officer (CNO). These pairs learn to develop a strong interpersonal relationship, as well as convey a vision of collaborative practice, which then serves as a role model for physician–nurse leadership pairs at lower levels. In many cases, the CMO and CNO offices are colocated next to each other; such physical proximity creates regular access to one another. These two individuals may also cochair clinical committees (e.g., critical care, patient safety, quality improvement) in which interprofessional collaboration is essential and in which the required collaboration can be visibly demonstrated to committee members. In these ways, the CMO and CNO can present a "united front" that establishes agendas and budgets for hospital and hospital system-wide efforts that implement collaboration from the top down. They can also send a consistent message to both medical and nursing personnel that their cooperation is important and expected. The dyads can further role model the importance of their collaboration in recruitment processes that stress teamwork.

As one illustration, the CMOs and CNOs of the component hospitals of the University of Pennsylvania Health System (UPHS) began to meet regularly in 2006 to create a shared voice for patient safety. This work resulted in the Blueprint for Quality and Patient Safety—the UPHS framework for clinical quality that is now in its third iteration. The report not only established physician- and nurse-sponsored goals but also created a vehicle for shared budgeting. Nurses and physicians no longer compete for resources to advance quality and safety. Instead, they work together in a way that enables them to negotiate with their fiscal partners with a united clinical voice (Robert Wood Johnson Foundation, 2015).

MICROSYSTEMS AND PATIENT INSTITUTES

Another recent approach to integrate the work of healthcare professionals is to reorganize it into multidisciplinary clusters at local levels in the institution to focus on specific patient subgroups. These have been alternatively labeled "clinical microsystems" (Nelson et al., 2002) and "patient institutes" (Porter & Teisberg, 2006). Such teams include physicians, nurses, pharmacists, social workers, and other ancillary professionals, all supported by information, technology, work processes, and other investments.

Based on the early work of Quinn (1992), these teams focus on and continually engineer the front-line relationships that apply the capabilities of the organization to meet the needs of its patients. Subsequent research examined the characteristics of these front-line teams that promoted quality of care (Mohr, 2000; Mohr, Batalden, & Barach, 2004; Barach & Johnson, 2006). These characteristics include leadership, information and information technology, interdependence (e.g., trust, collaboration, mutual support, recognition of others' roles), performance results and measurement, supportiveness of the larger health system, patient focus, staff focus (selective hiring), community and market focus, investment in process improvement, and investment in education training.

How do organizations transform professional work into such clinical microsystems of care? Much of this takes place via cross-training, team training, team building, and skill building in such areas as communication, leadership, and team performance evaluation with feedback. Perhaps more important is the careful selection (and self-selection) of professionals to join the microsystems. Such selection processes characterize the process of physician recruitment at some IDNs such as Kaiser and Geisinger. Microsystem success is probably driven as much by self-selection of team-oriented professionals as it is by all of the training cited above. Research evidence suggests that greater sharing of responsibility among physicians and nurses for cardiovascular care leads to increased structured delivery of chronic illness care (Nouwens, van Lieshout, van den Homberg, Laurant, & Wensing, 2014).

EFFORTS TO BREAK DOWN BOUNDARIES

Breaking down organizational boundaries and silos became a popular leadership strategy following the publicized effort of Jack Welch to (a) streamline the bloated workforce and bureaucracy at General Electric in the 1980s using the technique of "work-out" and (b) create a "boundaryless organization" (Ashkenas, Ulrich, Jick, & Kerr, 1995). It became institutionalized in the 1990s with executive efforts to "restructure and reengineer" their organization's processes (Hammer & Champy, 1994).

Healthcare organizations undertook their own version of reengineering during the 1990s. More recently, efforts similar to General Electric's work-out have been undertaken under the banner of "lean manufacturing" and the TPS. One common element to these undertakings is the joint participation of multiple professional groups in outlining the organization's key clinical processes. By doing so, the different professionals (a) learn how their colleagues view the work of the organization, (b) develop a shared understanding of how the work may be simplified, and (c) arrive at a mutually agreed on approach and timeline for implementing the needed changes. In this manner, professionals collaborate on system redesign to improve quality and/or efficiency.

To date, there is considerable anecdotal evidence on the implementation of the TPS at Virginia Mason Medical Center (VMMC). The results are impressive and encouraging to other hospitals thinking of adopting this approach. Nevertheless, after roughly 15 years of effort with TPS, there are no peer-reviewed empirical results of the success of TPS at VMMC. Indeed, meta-analyses suggest that TPS and lean manufacturing have not yet demonstrated their potential (Andersen, Rovik, & Ingebrigtsen, 2014). There is similarly meager support for the effects of restructuring and reengineering on hospital efficiency (Walston, Burns, & Kimberly, 2000).

Breaking down boundaries also entails conflict resolution approaches to deal with disputes in multidisciplinary teams. Such approaches are essential because conflict is inherent in teamwork. Research suggests that primary healthcare teams can invoke several strategies to resolve conflicts such as team leader interventions and conflict management protocols. Team individuals can further address conflict through strategies such as open and direct communication, humility, showing respect, and a willingness to find solutions (Brown et al., 2011).

Managing Healthcare Professionals and Preparing Them to Manage

Management involves the use of organizational tools and processes to help overcome fragmentation, increase coherence, and promote coordinated effort. These tools span the use of classic integrative devices (e.g., informal liaisons, formal integrators, cross-functional teams, matrix roles), older methods of unobtrusive control over professionals' decisions such as group practice norms and peer surveillance of physician errors (Freidson, 1975; Bosk, 1979), and newer ways to integrate professionals into bureaucracies (e.g., physician employment, integrated practice units). Healthcare professionals are not necessarily trained in the use and deployment of these tools and processes, however. Increasingly, professionals require training to prepare them to tackle the collaborative challenges described above.

COORDINATIVE DEVICES

Liaisons

Liaisons are perhaps the most rudimentary form of matrix organization designed to link together different functional specialties. They are informal, low-cost, and easy to both assemble and disassemble. They are also nonthreatening to existing professionals being linked because the liaisons have no formal authority and decision-making power.

The important role that patient liaisons can play has been recognized in clinical trials of care coordination (Peikes et al., 2009). Intense, face-to-face communication between patients and their providers is essential for those patients managing chronic illnesses. Such illnesses account for a disproportionate share of US healthcare spending and resist curative efforts. Instead, chronic care management requires an ongoing collaboration between patient and provider to monitor the patient's self-care behaviors, level of activation, care-seeking behaviors, and disease management. For such programs to work, physicians and nurses on hospital floors need to engage patients and liaisons to coordinate their joint care activities.

Formal Integrators

Organizations can take an additional step beyond liaison roles to coordinate functional specialties by installing formal integrator roles. Due to the growing interest in care coordination for elderly and chronically ill patients, hospitals have begun to hire full-time "care coordinators" to work with their physicians, nurses, and other professionals in both inpatient and outpatient clinics. Such personnel handle communications from patients, reduce gaps in communication and care among professionals on the care team, and facilitate patient transitions from the hospital to home or other care sites. Physicians perform similar roles on inpatient floors and in specialty areas (e.g., the intensive care unit) of the hospital. Nurse practitioners perform similar functions inside the offices of primary care physicians who have embraced PCMHs as their new organizational model of practice (Congressional Budget Office, 2012).

Because care coordinators work in a group and consultative context, it is difficult to evaluate the effectiveness of their particular role. Field studies evaluating their impact have identified various roles they play. These roles include having frequent face-to-face contact with patients (e.g., once a month), building strong rapport with patients' physicians through face-to-face contact at the hospital or medical office, using behavioral change techniques to help patients increase adherence to medications and self-care regimes, knowing when patients are hospitalized in order to provide support for care transitions to the home, acting as a communications hub among providers and between patient and providers, and having reliable information about patients' prescriptions and access to pharmacists or the medical director (Peikes et al., 2009; Brown, 2013).

There is a growing research base concerning the effectiveness of care coordination programs. To date, the results have been weak at best, largely due to the difficult task of coordinating care for the most expensive patient population—those with multiple chronic diseases (Congressional Budget Office, 2012; Brown, 2013). Problems identified include expectation of quick results, lack of provider incentives, and lack of data for providers on their own quality and efficiency.

Cross-functional Teams

Cross-functional teams are a major mode of coordinating activities of diverse practitioners. Such teams have been adopted as major vehicles for improving patient safety, quality, and care coordination in the form of care management teams (e.g., carveout programs for specific conditions, chronic care teams), PCMHs, and multi-specialty physician group practices.

Collaborative models to coordinate professional activities extend beyond physicians, administrators, and nurses. A growing number of health systems are recognizing the value of including other ancillary providers in care teams, such as pharmacists (Giberson, Yoder, & Lee, 2011). Pharmacists now round with physicians and residents in teaching hospitals to educate trainees about drug interactions, medication compliance, and drug utilization review. There is also growing recognition that more effective compliance with medication therapy can substitute for additional physician visits and hospitalizations, thereby lowering the total cost of care.

Research suggests that such collaborative teams are important but insufficient ingredients. These teams need to be *designed* to provide and coordinate patient-centered care. Three design elements are often mentioned: clear membership boundaries, interdependence that fosters collective responsibility for assessable outcomes (and incentives to induce this interdependence), and membership stability (Wageman, Hackman, & Lehman, 2005; Monroe-DeVita, Teague, & Moser, 2011). They must also have a patient focus, a clear statement of the team's purpose, a compelling direction, delegation of responsibility and control over their self-organization, and the infrastructure and resources needed to do their job (Wholey, Zhu, Knoke, Shah, & White, 2012).

Matrix Roles

Similar to the liaison and formal integrator roles, some organizations have developed executives with dual training in different professional worlds. Sociologists long ago referred to such individuals as "marginal men"—those suspended between two different cultures who lacked a clear identification with either, but who could import and export ideas and perspectives across disciplines and thereby break down organizational boundaries. Such marginal men personified organizational dyads inside the mind of one individual (Stonequist, 1937; Ziller, Stark, & Pruden, 1969).

The emergence of these boundary roles has been abetted by the growing desire of practicing physicians to diversify away from strictly clinical roles to occupy managerial roles in hospitals and other healthcare organizations. Part of this desire is driven by reimbursement pressures; part of it is driven by increasing practice workloads and regulatory burdens. Physicians are now attracted to become CMOs, chief medical informatics officers, leaders of quality management efforts, and academic department chairs in medical schools. Some physicians may occupy similar roles in managed care organizations. In growing recognition of this trend, the American College of Healthcare Executives has launched a "physician executives forum" that acknowledges the growing number and prominence of physicians in leadership roles overseeing healthcare provider organizations. Their effort was preceded by the formation of the American College of Physician Executives in 1975, which has since evolved to become the American Association of Physician Leadership, with its own journal (*Physician Leadership Journal*).

One spur to this movement has been the widely shared (but largely unsubstantiated) belief that physician executives can be more effective in managing a hospital medical staff and eliciting the cooperation of staff physicians. The logic here is that physician executives share the same professional degree and training as the staff physicians, share the same professional values such as clinical autonomy and patient focus, and speak the same language as the staff physicians. Continuing with this logic, there should thus be a higher potential for constructive dialogue and communication between administration and the medical staff, a greater degree of trust, and perhaps a greater ability to effectively work on organizational changes. As a result, physician executives may become more effective leaders of their organizations by virtue of bridging the traditional divide between the administrative hierarchy and the medical hierarchy.

First, there is no solid evidence that this bridging occurs easily or without conflict (Hoff, 1999). Second, there is no solid evidence that physician executives improve the leadership of hospital organizations or systems. Part of the problem is measurement: there are few physician CEOs of hospitals. According to one study, only 235 of the 6,500 US hospitals have such physician leadership (Gunderman & Kanter, 2009). There are some reports that hospitals with higher quality rankings are associated with physician leadership (Goodall, 2011; Parker-Pope, 2011). However, as Montgomery (2003) notes:

> It's very difficult to say how much of an organization's performance is affected by the fact that it has physicians in executive roles. Organizations seem to assume when they decide to bring physicians into high-level management positions that they need someone who will be a liaison to help articulate the organization's strategic direction and decisions to clinicians and communicate the views of clinicians back to management. That doesn't always work. A lot depends on the individual capabilities of the person in that role. We have some evidence that indicates that clinicians become quite distrustful of physicians who have gone over to the other side.
>
> We know from a number of case studies that people who are still on the clinical side aren't particularly happy dealing with those whom they now consider former colleagues. Much of that is a function of the individual and of the trustworthiness of the person in this very difficult hybrid professional position. Much depends on individual capabilities and interpersonal skills. Does the person act with integrity? Has the person demonstrated a history of competence as a physician as well as competence in management? It is an extremely difficult set of skills to maintain.

There is some recent evidence that the performance of such leadership roles may positively impact the job satisfaction of rank-and-file physicians underneath them and reduces their burnout (Shanafelt et al., 2015). Increased levels of leadership on the part of front-line physician supervisors (e.g., the ability to inform, engage, inspire, develop, and recognize) can increase physician satisfaction with work in the organization and decrease their level of emotional exhaustion and depersonalization. The findings reemphasize the importance of careful recruitment and selection of physician leaders.

PHYSICIAN EMPLOYMENT AND INTEGRATION MECHANISMS

Since the early 1990s, healthcare organizations have placed a major emphasis on "integration" with their professionals (particularly physicians). The integration movement was spawned by Medicare's Prospective Payment System of 1983, which altered the financial incentives for physicians and hospitals; hospitals were now paid a fixed rate based on the patients diagnosis-related group, or DRG, whereas physicians remained on fee-for-service reimbursement. Hospitals thus had an incentive to control spending, which physicians did not. To solve the issue of divergent incentives, hospitals sought to align their interests and goals with those of their medical staffs using a variety of mechanisms.

The Health Systems Integration Study (Shortell, Gillies, Anderson et al., 1993) developed a conceptual model that functional integration of administrative functions across hospitals within a system can foster physician–system economic integration (one component of which is employment), which in turn drives clinical integration (including coordination of care across professionals and sites of care). Some academic researchers (Shortell, Gillies, Anderson, Mitchell, & Morgan, 1993) and many executives believe that hospital employment of physicians can help foster greater collaboration of their organizations with physicians, as well as greater collaboration among clinicians to improve quality.

There is mixed evidence for these linkages at best (Burns & Muller, 2008). One reason is that clinical integration is much less well-developed than economic integration. Another reason is that the multiple vehicles of economic integration were never really designed to foster clinical integration and inter-professional collaboration. A third reason is that employed physicians have only slightly higher levels of organizational commitment compared to nonemployed physicians (Burns et al., 2001).

Additional research has identified three other mechanisms used by hospitals to integrate with physicians: noneconomic, economic, and clinical integration (Burns & Muller, 2008).

1. *Noneconomic integration* refers to hospitals' efforts to enlist physicians by making their facilities more attractive and accessible, their operations more efficient and convenient, their decision-making processes more participative and responsive, and their staffing better trained. These efforts can take the form of technology acquisitions, hospital branding, process flow

improvements, management information systems, physicians' liaisons, referral services, clinical councils, physician leadership development, medical staff development, and additions to the number and skill mix of the nursing staff.

2. *Economic integration* encompasses hospitals' provision of monetary payments to physicians to provide, manage, and/or improve clinical services and to perform organizational activities. These payments can take the form of professional service agreements, medical directorships, stipends, performance bonds, management contracts, gain sharing, leases, and co-management of clinical institutes and centers of excellence. Economic integration can also include joint investments (e.g., in medical office buildings, ambulatory surgery centers, diagnostic imaging centers, service lines, specialty hospitals) and joint-risk reimbursement contracts from payers (e.g., bundled payments, pay-for-performance, capitated risk).

3. *Clinical integration* refers to hospitals' structures and systems to coordinate patient care services across people, functions, activities, and sites over time. Common activities of clinical integration are utilization management programs, scheduling and registration systems, information systems that can track utilization by patient and provider, development of care standards, continuous quality improvement programs, clinical service lines, case management systems, population-based community health models, and disease and demand management systems.

Burns and Muller (2008) also examined the evidence base for these mechanisms (see Young, Charns, & Hereen, 2004). In general, most mechanisms either fail to increase integration or lack any substantiation; only a handful of mechanisms (e.g., bundled payment, concentration of inpatient activity at one hospital) actually served to increase integration of physicians with hospitals.

Some research studies examined mechanisms that increased physicians' collaboration with other professionals in the form of "care management practices" (CMPs). Shortell et al. (2001) found that the use of salary models for physicians was associated with both the comprehensiveness and deployment of CMPs. Rittenhouse et al. (2011) reported that hospital employment is associated with greater use of medical home processes. A review of the literature found few systematic effects of CMPs, however (Burns, Goldsmith, & Sen, 2013).

MANAGERIAL TRAINING

Several industry trade publications acknowledge hospitals' efforts to develop the management skills of local level managers and clinicians. Many of these skills are relevant to professional collaboration, including systems-based practice, interpersonal and communication skills, cross-disciplinary training, and multidisciplinary teams (Jarousse, 2015). Much of the training provided is on-the-job rather than through formal programs.

Over the past two or three decades, a host of formal management programs have been developed to train physicians, nurses (e.g., Johnson & Johnson Nursing Executives Program), and more recently care coordinators (e.g., Population Care Coordinator certificate program at Duke University). Only some of these programs are degree granting (e.g., offer an executive Master of Business Administration, or MBA). The goal is to supplement physicians' traditional clinical training with managerial training. Such training can include human resource management, financial management, strategic planning, information systems, and organizational design. More recently, medical schools have begun to introduce similar training into their four-year programs—but on a more limited basis. Medical school training can now include teamwork, system design, and insurance and reimbursement, for example.

The proliferation of management training programs has been occasioned by a proliferation in patient care sites (e.g., ambulatory surgery centers, free-standing diagnostic clinics, physician group practices, IPAs, and physician–hospital organizations). The growing entrepreneurial activity begs for greater managerial and financial skills to run these enterprises and also places a premium on skilled managers of ambulatory care sites, which are quite different than hospitals and nursing homes. Physicians are more attuned to retail care settings than are nonphysician managers of hospitals by virtue of their experience running community-based office practices.

How does such managerial training help resolve the paradox described above? Instead of or in addition to having physician executives at the top of the hierarchy, managerially trained and competent physicians at lower levels provide a cadre of "ambidextrous" professionals who may be better able to assume roles of "marginal men" operating at the boundary of clinician and managerial cultures. Physicians with both medical and managerial training can begin to balance these two different perspectives and hopefully offer synthetic solutions to difficult problems that harmonize both. Research evidence is sorely needed to verify this proposition.

UNOBTRUSIVE CONTROL OVER PROFESSIONAL DECISIONS

Finally, organizations can use a host of unobtrusive techniques to reorient the attitudes and behaviors of their professionals toward organizational goals such as collaboration and team-based practice. These techniques include peer pressure and report cards.

Use of Peer Pressure

Physicians and nurses are professionals who believe they should control the content of their own work (Freidson, 1988). Much of the supervision that professionals conduct with their own colleagues is through largely informal conversations that are horizontal and collegial, rather than through overt bureaucratic control. This is true of physicians more than it is for nurses. But, with the rise of ACOs and accountability for quality, there is greater impetus on the front-line care providers to hold each other responsible through peer pressure, informal feedback, and coaching. Thus, there is an institutional basis for stating that the main source of administration is peer pressure.

There are other reasons to suggest peer pressure as the foundation for managing the work of professionals. Research suggests that physicians have a hierarchy of loyalties (Sheldon, 1986). Their primary loyalty is to their patients. Then physicians are loyal to their immediate colleagues, whether those in their office practice or those in their specialty. Beyond that, physicians are loyal to their profession. Way beyond that, physicians are loyal to the institutions in which they practice. Patients do not exert peer pressure on physicians because of the large asymmetry in information between them. But colleagues who practice in proximity to physicians can and do exert peer pressure. Sociologists have argued this phenomenon operates by virtue of "practicing shoulder to shoulder" (i.e., by virtue of having colleagues observe what one does [Freidson, 1988]).

Among nurses, such peer pressure has been embedded in structured feedback sessions with peers as well as structured problem-focused discussions on difficult clinical issues. Some hospitals have also pursued peer accountability via "inter-assignment rounding," whereby nurses round with colleagues on patients outside of their individual direct care responsibility. Such mechanisms seek to promote collaboration within the medical and nursing hierarchies. Joint rounds between physicians, nurses, and pharmacists can likewise promote interdisciplinary collaboration.

Report Cards

The use of report cards represents an indirect form of exerting peer pressure. Report cards chart the professional's performance on various quality metrics (whether process or outcome measures) or utilization metrics (e.g., referrals or inpatient days per 1,000) relative to the clinician's peers. The names of the other clinicians may or may not be blinded, but the clinician knows where he or she stands in the distribution. It is common (but largely undocumented) wisdom that physicians do not like to be outliers at the lower end of the distribution relative to their peers. The use of the report cards thus serves as an impersonal way of encouraging clinicians to change their behaviors to conform—more like their peers higher up in the distribution.

Recent research suggests that report cards not only exert peer pressure but also intrinsic motivational effects (Kolstad, 2013). It is commonplace wisdom that physicians are driven to be the best and to do well as in the eyes of their patients. But what is less well known is that physicians can discover new information about themselves in published quality reports, which can motivate them to strive to provide better care. This is particularly true if the quality data reported about the physicians practice and that of others are risk-adjusted.

Collaborative Processes and Team Dynamics

In recent years, healthcare providers and researchers have turned their attention to cooperative processes to improve the care coordination and quality. As one illustration, these parties have formed several collaborative organizations to improve the delivery of care (e.g., the Institute for Healthcare Improvement, the Academic Innovations Collaborative). The Institute for Healthcare Improvement has formulated and disseminated best practices for providers who seek to achieve "the triple aim" (Berwick et al., 2008). The Academic Innovations Collaborative, which includes primary care practices, has conducted an evaluation of an initiative to improve team dynamics.

This research has identified many important components of collaborative practice, including trust, shared understanding, shared ambition (commitment), shared control, pursuit of mutual gains, accountability, communication and information exchange, development of relational capital, conflict resolution, and acting and feeling like a team (among others) (see Song et al., 2015; Valentijn et al., 2015). The limited findings to date suggest that such processes facilitate success with integrated care projects, care coordination, and clinical work satisfaction. These findings are consistent with prior research that team-based care (such as that found in PCMHs), often centered around nurse practitioners as care coordinators, promotes favorable patient experiences and quality outcomes (Jackson et al., 2013; Biernacki, Champagne, Peng, Maizel, & Turner, 2015).

Integrating Healthcare Delivery

The above review suggests some of the ways in which the broad forces of standardization, consumerism, innovation, and competition call for greater collaboration among professionals, but also run counter to the tenets of professionalism—and thus make it difficult to achieve the desired collaboration. The push for *standardization* has been fueled by the call to reduce clinician errors, to reduce practice variations, to reduce waste and patient waiting times, and to increase value (e.g., by achieving stipulated quality metrics). These have placed a premium on improving patient experience, increasing patient safety, improving care transitions and patient handoffs, increasing patient flow and convenience, and demonstrating value. The push for *consumerism* has likewise been fueled by the call to reduce waste but also by the need to increase patients' engagement in their own care (e.g., self-care), with the clinician teams tending to them, and with the cost and quality of the care they seek. The push for *innovation* has been fueled by the need to develop better treatment approaches to contain the costs of chronic care, to seek out more cost-effective and convenient sites of care (e.g., retail clinics, medical homes), and the need to embed clinical knowledge in information technology systems to help clinicians select care approaches and communicate with one another. The impact of such innovation has been the recognition that nonphysician professionals (e.g., nurse practitioners, pharmacists, patient liaisons, care coordinators) may play a greater role in both inpatient and ambulatory care. Finally, the rise of *competition* between physicians and hospitals since the 1980s has occasioned the situation where the two most important and expensive actors in the healthcare system both collaborate and compete with one another in the care continuum. Hospitals are thus not only trying to partner with physicians (e.g., to run centers of clinical excellence) but also trying to employ them. They are thus at the center of efforts to develop leadership and managerial approaches to resolve the conflict between collaboration and professionalism noted at the outset of this chapter.

As far as "integrated care" is concerned, this implies that it is insufficient to merely implement new standards, customer orientations, or innovation systems. Attempts to "integrate" services in such instrumental ways will not improve collaborative capacity. On the contrary, it will strengthen the paradoxes of effectively improving healthcare described above. Instead of optimizing systems, leadership and management are ideally (re)working cultures, boundaries, and values so that more appropriate incentives are established to actually adapt ways of working.

These practical developments can be linked to more academic reflections on changing medical professionalism. Instead of seeing medical professional action as matter of subdividing work domains and isolating jurisdictions from outside worlds, with strict boundaries and autonomies, service delivery must be seen as a matter of integrating these domains, and professionalism must be seen as a matter of establishing *connections* between the various segments that make up healthcare (e.g., Noordegraaf, 2015). Instead of seeing physicians, nurses, therapists, and so on, as working within separate work domains that regulate themselves, medical action cuts across domains and involves all of these workers; they are jointly responsible for delivering care. Healthcare delivery calls for institutionalized, directed, and well-organized medical processes that combine the actions of multiple workers. These processes generate valuable outcomes that are not so much production outcomes with clear monetary value as productive outcomes with public value. Integrated healthcare delivery takes place on the right scale, is state-of-the-art, is efficient, solves problems, serves society, and is legitimate.

This explains our earlier emphasis on (a) leadership as a matter of institutions and values and (b) management as a matter of coordinating work forces. Medical work has to be coordinated on a daily basis, but such work must now occur within a broader context of improved value along a number of dimensions (quality, safety, budgetary, and innovation) in the eyes of multiple stakeholders (professionals, payers, and patients). This implies that integration is no mere functional or instrumental affair. More than just using the proper procedures and optimizing the right systems, integrated care calls for a combination of the technical "heart" of professional work—the right rules, incentives, cultures (most specifically collaborative cultures), and patient orientation. In addition, healthcare professionals can no longer focus on single cases and the treatment of individual patients; now they are increasingly called on to focus on the health of populations—even if the economic incentive or financial upside to do so is small. Healthcare professionals have become responsible for *co-organizing* healthcare among themselves as well as with patients and other stakeholders. Taking up such responsibility leads to cultural frictions, because—as we argued—different ways of knowing, being, and acting are at stake. This requires that leading and managing also become part of medical work (e.g., Kirkpatrick & Noordegraaf 2015; Noordegraaf, 2015) in order to overcome these cultural frictions. The following section explores the practical and theoretical implications that flow from this view.

Implications

PRACTICAL CONSIDERATIONS

The move toward more integrated care can be seen as a cultural transition. Moving beyond the various obstacles to collaboration and divisive forces affect ways of being, knowing, and acting. This implies that healthcare professionals and their organizations must invest in the development of new capabilities.

First, they will have to strengthen leadership and management *competencies* that allow professionals to deal with the many challenges facing healthcare delivery (e.g., reducing medical errors, promoting patient safety, and reducing levels of spending). There are increasing signs that key players now take this seriously and are undertaking the needed educational and organizational adaptations. These adaptations are not solely about "grand" leadership development, including the production of organizational leaders, but also about turning physicians into operational or "front-line leaders." Blumenthal, Bernard, Bohnen, & Bohmer (2012) argue that "... effective frontline clinical leadership improves both clinical outcomes and satisfaction for patients and providers" (p. 514). They even stress there is a "leadership gap" (p. 515)—too much focus on organizational leaders and too little stress on leadership development within medical work forces. Teams of medical workers require competencies such as "communication, team building, planning and priority setting, assessing performance, problem solving and leading" (p. 515).

Second and related, it is important to focus on the *education* and (thus) the *socialization* of future healthcare professionals. In many ways this is a fundamental shift, as physicians acquire a clinical "habitus" that determines how to view the world—in fact, how they distinguish themselves from the rest of the world (e.g., Witman, Schmid, Meurs, & Wilems, 2008). In some ways this is a practical shift, connecting the "clinical gaze" to other and outside worlds. This can be done, at least partly, by establishing curriculum changes in medical schools aimed at developing competencies to work in teams, dealing with patient- and stakeholder-orientations, becoming accountable for actions, and spanning boundaries. Such competencies might become part of new professional repertoires (see Blumenthal et al., 2012) that enable medical professionals to develop "connective professionalism" (see Noordegraaf, 2015). New competency frameworks such as the CanMEDS model developed in Canada (Frank, 2005) and used in other Western countries exemplify this development by stressing the need of communicative, collaborative, and managerial/leadership competencies of physicians. Newer frameworks seek to move beyond development of individual competencies and inculcate situational approaches for establishing more integrated medical care. Entrustable professional activities (EPAs), for example, are used to implement a more integrated view of medical action (e.g., Hauer et al., 2013; Ten Cate, 2014). In order to behave competently, physicians and other medical workers need to apply multiple competencies in the light of real-life clinical situations. EPAs are "units of professional practice, defined as tasks or responsibilities to be entrusted to the unsupervised execution by a trainee once he or she has attained sufficient specific competence" (Ten Cate, 2013, p. 157). This represents a cultural transition as physicians are taught how to become more dependent instead of "autonomous" workers.

Finally, it is important to pay attention to broader forms of *organization development*, which also aim to strengthen the work cultures and systems within healthcare organizations. Even when leadership is improved and medical workers are better trained, other conditions help to enhance collaborative capacity. As collaboration calls for overcoming structural boundaries (including socialization, interests, reputations, and status), organizational cultures, systems, and incentives can make or break sound professional processes. More integrated medical work might be hard to attain when budgetary incentives are lacking, when performance systems do not match collaborative ambitions, or when innovators are not supported. For example, Reay and Hinings (2009) stress the importance of organizational mechanisms for improving "pragmatic collaboration" between organizational and professional actors, within healthcare. They show how physicians can be connected to organizational decision-making as experts, how they can be tied to organizational processes in more informal ways, and how spaces for joint innovation might be created.

THEORETICAL CONSIDERATIONS

The foregoing suggests the following theoretical implications. First and foremost, we need better understandings of changing forms of *professionalism* and *professional action*. As argued, well-led and well-managed medical work and integrated care go against traditional images of autonomous professionals who treat individual cases as effectively as possible. Instead of repeating such classic images and ideals, it will be more fruitful to focus on the "hybridization" of medical service delivery (e.g., Empson et al., 2015). Whereas medical professionalism used to be seen as a rather "pure" type, as exemplified by Freidson's depiction at the start of our chapter, professionalism has turned into a "mutated" phenomenon (Adler & Kwon, 2013). From a more positive point of view, professionalism has turned into a hybrid phenomenon in which its classic components—professional ethos, moral stature, technical skills, and case-orientation—are combined with new components such as organizational awareness, political sensitivity, and stakeholder connections. The latter components signify the rise of more connective forms of professionalism (e.g., Kirkpatrick & Noordegraaf, 2015; Noordegraaf, 2015) in which the autonomies of different professionals do not oppose or work against one another but rather interrelate to and support one another.

Furthermore, we need more insight into the *conditions* and *mechanisms* that contribute to the rise of collaborative care. Under which conditions are certain means and mechanisms for leading and managing healthcare workers more or less effective? In addition, we need more insight into the *effects* that these new approaches have, as far as "effectiveness" is concerned. Healthcare effects are more than pure medical outcomes and quality of care. They include effects upon patients and workers themselves, including worker wellbeing, commitment, vitality, stress, and burnout. They also encompass broader societal impacts including productivity, gross domestic product growth, and population health. According to modern management perspectives, this is a matter realizing *public value* (e.g., Moore, 1995). Healthcare service delivery generates value conflicts; medical action and medical systems must be able to cope with multiple values.

In order to study *public value creation*, we require additional insight, inter alia, in how medical competency is actually developed—whether and how medical workers develop the ability to manage multiple value needs and expectations. As argued, it is more than enhancing separate competencies "within" workers and more about entrusting medical workers with real-life situations, which call for joint efforts. It is about the day-to-day usage of medical standards, protocols, and routines against institutional and stakeholder backgrounds.

Conclusions and Ways Forward

Changes in healthcare contexts demand more seamless and integrated care, higher value to patients and payers, and satisfaction of multiple stakeholders' expectations. These very same changes, however, also pressure providers and generate divisions among them. Traditionally in the face of pressures, boundaries between medical groups were reinforced, new tasks and standards were kept at a distance, and new professional groups and interventions faced resistance. Going forward, healthcare providers will have to lead and manage their professionals in new ways to promote integration.

We have sketched several practical ways to lead and manage healthcare. The goal is to improve (a) connections among the professionals delivering healthcare; (b) administrative, managerial and operational processes; and (c) services to patients and stakeholders. We have also discussed broader practical and theoretical implications. Instead of focusing on the *old* professionalism, which involves individual professionals treating cases, we have to focus on the *new* professionalism, which involves groups of professionals, semiprofessionals, and other workers coorganizing sound medical processes, serving multiple patients and stakeholders, and improving the health of populations. This is neither tightly controlled from above nor loosely linked to bottom-up actions. It is possible to secure links between occupational and organizational logics, especially when leadership capabilities are enhanced, medical workers are educated and trained in new ways, and when organizational conditions and climates facilitate the rise of collaborative care. Sound institutions, public values, competent work forces, and coordinated work *together* comprise integrated care and enable us to move beyond the paradoxes of leading and managing healthcare.

References

Abbott, A. (1988). *The system of professions: An essay on the division of expert labor.* Chicago, IL: University of Chicago Press.

Adler, P. S., & Kwon, S. W. (2013). The mutation of professionalism as a contested diffusion process: Clinical guidelines as carriers of institutional change in medicine. *Journal of Management Studies, 50*(5), 930–962.

Adler, P. S., Kwon, S. W., & Heckscher, C. (2008). Perspective-professional work: The emergence of collaborative community. *Organization Science, 19*(2), 359–376.

Andersen, H., Rovik, K. A., & Ingebrigtsen, T. (2014). Lean thinking in hospitals: Is there a cure for the absence of evidence? A systematic review of reviews. *BMJ Open 2014, 4*, e003873. doi:10.1136/bmjopen-2013-003873.

Ashkenas, R., Ulrich, D., Jick, T., & Kerr, S. (1995). *The boundaryless organization.* San Francisco, CA: Jossey-Bass.

Barach, P., & Johnson, J. K. (2006). Understanding the complexity of redesigning care around the clinical microsystem. *Quality & Safety in Health Care, 15* Suppl 1, i10–6. doi:15/suppl_1/i10 [pii].

Berwick, D. M., Nolan, T. W., & Whittington, J. (2008). The triple aim: Care, health, and cost. *Health Affairs, 27*(3), 759–769.

Biernacki, P. J., Champagne, M. T., Peng, S., Maizel, D. R., & Turner, B. S. (2015). Transformation of care: Integrating the registered nurse care coordinator into the patient-centered medical home. *Population Health Management, 18*(5), 330–336.

Blumenthal, D. M., Bernard, K., Bohnen, J., & Bohmer, R. (2012). Addressing the leadership gap in medicine: residents' need for systematic leadership development training. *Academic Medicine: Journal of the Association of American Medical Colleges, 87*(4), 513–522.

Boev, C., & Xia, Y. (2015). Nurse-physician collaboration and hospital-acquired infections in critical care. *Critical Care Nurse, 35*(2), 66–72.

Bohmer, R. M. J., & Ferlins, E. M. (2008). *Virginia Mason Medical Center.* Harvard case study. 9-606-044.

Bosk, C. (1979). *Forgive and remember: Managing medical failure.* Chicago, IL: University of Chicago Press.

Brint, S. G. (2006). Saving the "Soul of Professionalism": Freidson's institutional ethics and the defense of professional autonomy. *Knowledge, Work and Society, 4*(2), 101–129.

Brown, J., Lewis, L., Ellis, K., Stewart, M., Freeman, T. R., & Kasperski, M. J. (2011). Conflict on interprofessional primary health care teams—can it be resolved? *Journal of Interprofessional Care, 25*, 4–10.

Brown, R. (2013). Lessons from the past for Medicare reforms under the ACA: Improving care for high-need beneficiaries. Presentation to AcademyHealth (Baltimore, MD).

Bucher, R., & Strauss, A. (1961). Professions in process. *American Journal of Sociology, 66*, 325–334.

Buerki, R., & Vottero, L. (2002). *The profession of pharmacy and pharmaceutical care.* In K. H. Calvin & R. P. Penna (Eds.), *Pharmaceutical care: A Primer on the pharmacist's changing role in patient care.* (pp. 3–17). American Society of Health-System Pharmacists.

Bunderson, J., Lofstrom, S., & Van de Ven, A. (1998). Allina Medical Group: A division of Allina Health System. In P. M. Ginter, L. M. Swayne, & W. J. Duncan (Eds.), *Strategic management of health care organizations,* (3rd ed.) (pp. 602–619). Malden, MA: Blackwell Publishers.

Burns, J. M. (1978). *Leadership.* New York, NY: Harper Collins.

Burns, L. R., Alexander, J. A., Shortell, S. M., Zuckerman, H. S., Budetti, P. P., Gillies, R. R., & Waters, T. M. (2001). Physician commitment to organized delivery systems. *Medical Care, 39*(7), I-9-I-29.

Burns, L. R., & Becker, S. (1987). Leadership and managership. In S. Shortell & A. Kaluzny (Eds.), *Health care management: A text in organizational theory and behavior*, (2nd edition) (147–186) John Wiley & Sons.

Burns, L. R., David, G., & Helmchen, L. A. (2011). Strategic response by providers to specialty hospitals, ambulatory surgery centers, and retail clinics. *Population Health Management*, *14*(2), 69–77.

Burns, L. R., Goldsmith, J. C., & Sen, A. (2013). Horizontal and vertical integration of physicians: A tale of two tails. In J. Goes, G. T. Savage, & L. Friedman (Eds.), Annual Review of Health Care Management: Revisiting the Evolution of Health Systems Organization. *Advances in Health Care Management*, *15*, 39–118.

Burns, L. R., & Muller, R. W. (2008). Hospital-physician collaboration: Landscape of economic integration and impact on clinical integration. *Milbank Quarterly*, *86*(3), 375–434.

Chandler, A. (1977). *The visible hand: The managerial revolution in American business* Cambridge, MA: Harvard University Press.

Charns, M. P., & Tewksbury, L. J. S. (1993). *Collaborative management in health care*. San Francisco, CA: Jossey-Bass.

Congressional Budget Office. (2012). *Lessons from Medicare's demonstration projects on disease management, care coordination, and value-based payment*. Washington, DC: Congressional Budget Office.

Crosson, F. J. (2009). 21st-century health care—the case for integrated delivery systems. *New England Journal of Medicine, 361*(14), 1324–1325.

Eisenberg, J. M. (1986). *Doctors' decisions and the cost of medical care*. Ann Arbor, MI: Health Administration Press.

Eisenberg, J. (2002). Physician utilization: The state of research about physicians' practice patterns. *Medical Care, 40*(11), 1016–1035.

Elhauge, E. (2010). *The fragmentation of US health care: causes and solutions*. New York, NY: Oxford University Press.

Empson, L., Muzio, D., Broschak, J., & Hinings, B. (2015). *Oxford handbook of professional service firms*. Oxford, UK: Oxford University Press.

Frank, J. R. (2005). *The CanMEDS 2005 physician competency framework: Better standards, better physicians, better care*. Ottawa, Canada: Royal College of Physicians and Surgeons of Canada.

Freidson, E. (1975). *Doctoring together: A study of professional social control*. Chicago, IL: University of Chicago Press.

Freidson, E. (1988). *Profession of medicine: A study of the sociology of applied knowledge*. Chicago, IL: University of Chicago Press.

Freidson, E. (2001). *Professionalism: The third logic*. Cambridge, UK: Polity Press.

Giberson, S., Yoder, S., & Lee, M. P. (2011). *Improving patient and health system outcomes through advanced pharmacy practice. A report to the U.S. Surgeon General*. Office of the Chief Pharmacist. U.S. Public Health Service. Retrieved from http://www.accp.com/docs/positions/misc/improving_patient_and_health_system_outcomes.pdf

Goodall, A. H. (2011). Physician-leaders and hospital performance: is there an association? *Social Science & Medicine, 73*(4), 535–539.

Gunderman, R., & Kanter, S. L. (2009). Perspective: Educating physicians to lead hospitals. *Academic Medicine: Journal of the Association of American Medical Colleges, 84*(10), 1348–1351. doi:10.1097/ACM.0b013e3181b6eb42 [doi].

Ham, C., Imison, C., Goodwin, N., Dixon, A., & South, P. (2011). Where next for the NHS reforms? The case for integrated care. *The King's Fund* (London, UK: The King's Fund).

Hammer, M., & Champy. J. (1994). *Reengineering the corporation: A manifesto for business revolution*. New York, NY: HarperCollins Publishers.

Hauer, K., Soni, K., Cornett, P., et al. (2013). Developing entrustable professional activities as the basis for assessment of competence in an internal medicine residency: A feasibility study. *Journal of General Internal Medicine, 28*(8), 1110–1114.

Hoff, T. (1999). The social organization of physician managers in a changing HMO. *Work and Occupations, 26*(3), 324–351.

Hoff, T. (2013). Embracing a diversified future for US primary care. *The American Journal of Managed Care, 19*(1), e9–e13.

Hood, L. (2014). *Leddy and Pepper's conceptual bases of professional nursing.* (8th ed.). Baltimore, MD: Lippincott Williams & Wilkins.

Institute of Medicine. (2011). *The Future of Nursing: Leading Change, Advancing Health.* (Washington, DC: National Academies Press).

Jackson, G. L., Powers, B. J., Chatterjee, R., et al. (2013).Improving patient care: The patient centered medical home. A systematic review. *Annals of Internal Medicine, 158*(3), 169–178.

Jackson Healthcare. (2015). *Filling the Void: 2013 Physician Outlook and Practice Trends.*

Jarousse, L. A. (April 14, 2015). Developing physician leaders. *Hospitals and Health Networks.* Retrieved from http://www.hhnmag.com/articles/2974-hospitals-find-health-it-help-in-their-own-backyards.

Jauhar, S. (August 29, 2014). Why doctors are sick of their profession. *Wall Street Journal.* Retrieved from http://www.wsj.com/articles/the-u-s-s-ailing-medical-system-a-doctors-perspective-1409325361.

Kirkpatrick, I., & Noordegraaf, M. (2015). Hybrid professionalism: The re-shaping of occupational and organisational logics. In L. Empson, D. Muzio, J. Broschak & B. Hinings (Eds.), *The Oxford handbook on professional service firms,* 92–112. Oxford, UK: Oxford University Press.

Kolstad, J. (2013). Information and quality when motivation is intrinsic: Evidence from surgeon report cards. *American Economic Review, 103*(7), 2875–2910.

Lawrence, P. R., & Lorsch, J. (1967). *Organizations and environment: Managing differentiation and integration.* Reading, MA: Harvard Business School.

Lehman, E. (1975). *Coordinating health care: Explorations in interorganizational relations.* Beverly Hills, CA: Sage Publications.

Leistikow, I. P., Kalkman, C. J., & de Bruijn, H. (2011). Why patient safety is such a tough nut to crack. *BMJ (Clinical Research Ed.), 342,* d3447. doi:10.1136/bmj.d3447 [doi].

Martin, G., Currie, G., & Finn, R. (2009). Reconfiguring or reproducing intra-professional boundaries? Specialist expertise, generalist knowledge and the "modernization"of the medical workforce. *Social Science & Medicine, 68*(7), 1191–1198.

Mehrotra, A., Epstein, A. M., & Rosenthal, M. B. (2006). Do integrated medical groups provide higher-quality medical care than individual practice associations? *Annals of Internal Medicine, 145,* 826–833.

Mintzberg, H. (2012). Managing the myths of health care. *World Hospitals and Health Services, 48*(3), 05.

Mohr, J. (2000). *Forming, operating, and improving microsystems of care.* Hanover, NH: Center for the Evaluative Clinical Sciences, Dartmouth College.

Mohr, J., Batalden, P., & Barach, P. (2004). Integrating patient safety into the clinical microsystem. *Quality Safety Health Care, 13*(Suppl. II), ii34–ii38.

Monroe-DeVita, M., Teague, G. B., & Moser, L. L. (2011). The TMACT: A new tool for measuring fidelity to assertive community treatment. *Journal of American Psychiatric Nurses Association, 17*(1), 17–29.

Montgomery, K. (November 2003). Physician executives need not fly blind. *Managed Care.* Retrieved from http://www.managedcaremag.com/archives/0311/0311.qna_montgomery.html.

Moore, M. H. (1995). *Creating public value: Strategic management in government.* Cambridge, MA: Harvard University Press.

Moses, H., Matheson, D. H. M., Dorsey, E. R., George, B. P., Sadoff, D., & Yoshimura, S. (2013). The anatomy of health care in the United States. *Journal of the American Medical Association, 310*(18), 1947–1964.

Naymik, M. (July 22, 2009). President Barack Obama's Cleveland Clinic visit highlights role model of health care. Retrieved from http://blog.cleveland.com/metro/2009/07/president_barack_obamas_visit.html.

Nelson, E. C., Batalden, P. B, Huber, T. P., Moher, J. J., Godfrey, M. M., Headrick, L. A., & Wasson, J. H. (2002). Microsystems in health care: Part 1. Learning from high-performing front-line clinical units. *Joint Commission Journal of Quality Improvement, 28*(9), 472–493.

Noordegraaf, M. (2011). Risky business: How professionals and professionals fields (must) deal with organizational issues. *Organization Studies, 32*(10), 1349–1371.

Noordegraaf, M. (2015). Hybridity and beyond: (new) forms of professionalism in changing organizational and societal contexts. *Journal of Professions and Organizations, 2*(2), 187–206.

Nouwens, E., van Lieshout, J., van den Homberg, P., Laurant, M., & Wensing, M. (2014). Shifting cardiovascular care to nurses results in structured chronic care. *American Journal of Managed Care, 20*(7), 278–284.

Parker-Pope, T. (September 14, 2011). It's not discipline, it's a teachable moment. *The New York Times.* Retrieved from http://www.nytimes.com/2008/09/15/health/healthspecial2/15discipline.html.

Pauly, M., & Redisch, M. (1973). The not-for-profit hospital as a physicians' cooperative. *The American Economic Review, 63*(1), 87–99.

Peikes, D., Chen, A., Schore, J., & Brown, R. (2009). Effects of care coordination on hospitalization, quality of care, and health care expenditures among Medicare beneficiaries: 15 randomized trials. *Journal of the American Medical Association, 301*(6), 603–618.

Plochg, T., Klazinga, N., & Starfield, B. (2009). Transforming medical professionalism to fit changing health needs. *BMC Medicine, 7*(64).

Porter, M. E., & Teisberg, E. O. (2006). *Redefining health care: Creating value-based competition on results.* Boston, MA: Harvard Business School Publishing.

Quinn, J. B. (1992). *Intelligent enterprise: A knowledge and service based paradigm for industry.* New York, NY: The Free Press.

Reay, T., & Hinings, C. R. (2009). Managing the rivalry of competing institutional logics. *Organization Studies, 30*(6), 629–652.

Rittenhouse, D. R., Casalino, L. P., Shortell, S. M., McClellan, S. R., Gillies, R. R., Alexander, J. A., & Drum, M. L. (2011). Small and medium-size physician practices use few patient-centered medical home processes, *Health Affairs, 30*(8), 1575–1584.

Robert Wood Johnson Foundation. (2015). *Promising Interprofessional Collaboration Practices: Lessons from the Field*. Princeton, NJ: The Robert Wood Johnson Foundation.

Rousseau, D. M. (1990). New hire perceptions of their own and their employer's obligations: A study of psychological contracts. *Journal of Organizational Behavior, 11*(5), 389–400.

Ryan, J., Doty, M., Hamel, L., Norton, M., Abrams, M. K., & Brodie, M. (August 5, 2015). Primary care providers' views of recent trends in health care delivery and payment. *The Commonwealth Fund*. Retrieved from http://www.commonwealthfund.org/publications/issue-briefs/2015/aug/primary-care-providers-views-delivery-payment.

Sager, A., & Socolar, D. (2005). Health costs absorb one-quarter of economic growth, 2000-2005. *Physician for A National Health Program*. Retrieved from http://www.pnhp.org/news/2005/february/health-costs-absorb-one-quarter-of-economic-growth.

Scott, W. R., Ruef, M., Mendel, P. J., & Caronna, C. A. (2000). *Institutional change and health-care organizations: From professional dominance to managed care*. Chicago, IL: University of Chicago Press.

Selznick, P. (1957). *Leadership in administration*. Berkeley, CA: University of California Press.

Shanafelt T. D., Boone S., Tan L., et al. (2012). Burnout and satisfaction with work-life balance among US physicians relative to the general US population. *Archives of Internal Medicine, 172*, 1377–1385.

Shanafelt, T. D., Gorringe, G., Menaker, R., et al. (2015). Impact of organizational leadership on physician burnout and satisfaction. *Mayo Clinic Proceedings, 90*(4), 432–440.

Sheldon, A. (1986). *Managing doctors*. Washington DC: Beard Books.

Shortell, S. M., Gillies, R. R., Anderson, D. A., Mitchell, J. B., & Morgan, K. L. (1993). Creating organized delivery systems: The barriers and facilitators. *Hospital & Health Services Administration, 38*, 447–466.

Shortell, S. M., Zazzali, J., Burns, L. R., et al. (2001). Implementing evidence-based medicine: The role of market pressures, compensation incentives, and culture in physician organizations. *Medical Care, 39*(7), 162–178.

Song, H., Ryan, M., Tendulkar, S., et al. (2015). Team dynamics, clinical work satisfaction, and patient care coordination between primary care providers: A mixed methods study. *Health care management review*.

Stonequist, E. V. (1937). *Marginal man: A study in personality and culture conflict*. New York, NY: Russell and Russell.

Sutcliffe, K. M. (2011). High reliability organizations (HROs). *Best Practice & Research Clinical Anaesthesiology, 25*(2), 133–144.

Ten Cate, O. (2013). Nuts and bolts of entrustable professional activities. *Journal of Graduate Medical Education, 5*(1), 157–158.

Ten Cate, O. (2014). AM Last page: What entrustable professional activities add to a competency-based curriculum. *Academic Medicine, 98*(4), 691.

Valentijn, P. P., Ruwaard, D., Vrijhoef, H. J., de Bont, A., Arends, R. Y., & Bruijnzeels, M. A. (2015). Collaboration processes and perceived effectiveness of integrated care projects in primary care: a longitudinal mixed-methods study. *BMC health services research, 15*(1), 1.

Vize, R. (2012). Integrated care: a story of hard won success. *BMJ (Clinical Research Ed.), 344,* e3529. doi:10.1136/bmj.e3529 [doi].

Vogus, T. J., Sutcliffe, K. M., & Weick, K. E. (2010). Doing no harm: enabling, enacting, and elaborating a culture of safety in health care. *The Academy of Management Perspectives, 24*(4), 60–77.

Wageman, R., Hackman, J. R., & Lehman, E. (2005). Team diagnostic survey: Development of an instrument. *Journal of Applied Behavioral Science, 41*(4), 373–398.

Walston, S., Burns, L. R., & Kimberly, J. (2000). Does reengineering really work? An examination of the context and outcomes of hospital reengineering programs. *Health Services Research, 34*(6), 1363–1388.

Weinberg, D. B., Cooney-Miner, D., Perloff, J. N., Babington, L., & Avgar, A. C. (2011). Building collaborative capacity: Promoting interdisciplinary teamwork in the absence of formal teams. *Medical Care, 49*(8), 716–723.

Wholey, D. R., Zhu, X., Knoke, D., Shah, P., & White, K. M. (2012). Managing to care: Design and implementation of patient-centered care management teams. In S. Mick & D. Goldberg (Eds.), *Advances in Health Care Organization Theory,* (2nd Edition). San Francisco, CA: Jossey-Bass.

Witman, Y., Schmid, G. A. C., Meurs, P., & Wilems, D. L. (2008). Doctors in the lead: Balancing between two worlds. *Organization, 18*(4), 477–495.

Wynd, C. A. (2003). Current factors contributing to professionalism in nursing. *Journal of Professional Nursing, 19*(5), 251–261.

Young, G. J., Charns, M. P., & Hereen, T. C. (2004). Product line management in professional organizations: An empirical test of competing theoretical perspectives. *Academy of Management Journal, 47*(5), 723–734.

Ziller, R. C., Stark, B. J., & Pruden, H. O. (1969). Marginality and integrative management positions. *Academy of Management Journal, 12*(4), 487–495.

Zismer, D. K., Brueggemann, J., & James, M. D. (2010). Examining the "dyad" as a management model in integrated health systems. *Physician Executive Journal, 36*(1), 14–19.

COMMENTARY TO ACCOMPANY CHAPTER 5

Ralph W. Muller

THIS COMPREHENSIVE AND sweeping review by Noordegraaf and Burns appropriately focuses on one of the most significant challenges in healthcare today. This issue involves reconciling physician professionalism with the signals from (a) the payers of healthcare for more cost accountability and (b) the patients/consumers for more coordination of their care. As the authors describe, physicians are at the core of the healthcare system but are not as responsive to these signals as the other "actors" in the system want them to be. Thus, for example, hospitals, insurers, and governmental policymakers are taking measures to try to coordinate delivery of care (e.g., health reform, integrated delivery networks, value-based purchasing, and payment bundles). And with the rise of consumerism, abetted by changes in technology (e.g., the Internet, mobile technology), patients are collectively prompting innovation to make healthcare more patient-centered.

This changing healthcare context is making new demands on providers. Physicians and non-physician medical professionals are being asked to behave differently from what they have been trained and what they have done for many years. Physicians as professionals have traditionally relied on specialized knowledge as their main function; their new role calls for increased care standardization. There is strong evidence that variations in care both at the broad regional level and within healthcare organizations lead to worse outcomes and increased errors. Just as manufacturers reached similar conclusions in the last century, physicians need to balance professional specialized knowledge with the benefits of efficient delivery of care that results from "routinizing" care processes.

This review focuses on another key issue in healthcare, which is how to organize and lead healthcare professionals to produce high-quality, cost-effective care. The Affordable Care Act, in contrast to the managed care movement of the 1990s, puts providers in the central role of how to organize themselves to achieve this goal. The challenge is that many provider-based organizations do not have experience managing healthcare professionals in multidisciplinary teams to achieve high-quality, low-cost care across the continuum (e.g., physicians largely acted as their own independent agents; physician employment is a relatively recent phenomenon for most healthcare organizations). Also, few organizations have experience in managing care outside their organizational borders, whether it is with other hospitals, physician groups, postacute facilities, or systems for home care, which brings a host of new challenges in managing patients across the continuum. The positive evidence from some health systems that do manage care across the continuum (e.g., Kaiser Permanente, Mayo Clinic) likely result in part from self-selection of physicians into these organizations, whereby autonomizers are less likely to join, so extrapolating their results to a broader population may be problematic.

Most stakeholders agree that physicians and non-physician medical professionals need to work in a more team-based, coordinated way to produce higher quality, more efficient care across the care continuum. What is less clear is how to execute on this vision. Saying we want to achieve the "triple aim" of better quality, more access, and lower cost is not a road map for doing so. New organizing models are essential for achieving this care integration. The authors identify many forces that must be overcome to better coordinate care, including technical, functional, moral, political, and cultural. They also identify multiple models that are being used to overcome these barriers—physician and executive dyads, physician and nurse dyads, microsystems, and patient institutes—and other coordinating roles such as liaisons, care managers, and matrix roles such as physician executives. It is unlikely that there will be one dominant model; instead, the organizing and coordinating model must align with the broader organizational culture and healthcare organization structure. More evidence on the effectiveness of these various models is needed.

So how do we transition to this new collaborative care model? As the authors argue, the medical profession must accommodate these signals into their values and work. Multidisciplinary teams and providing care across patient settings require leadership and management, particularly to overcome the fragmentation that has traditionally existed in healthcare. The leaders of healthcare systems, whether they are physicians or for most of them, trained in other fields, must shape the culture to value these demands from payers, policymakers and patients, and teach the team of caregivers, not just physicians, how to adapt. They must also be present at all levels of the organization not only in promoting collaboration but in the alignment of roles, incentives, and goals.

The managerial structure of these systems also has to accommodate these signals into their daily processes and do the hard work of changing healthcare delivery at the front line of care—that is, where the patient experiences it. The authors appropriately note that many of the remedies suggested in the policy and managerial literature lack evidence of effectiveness. Simple fixes rarely work, as they note, and those of us in managerial roles should proceed in the course they recommend: integrating these signals from outside into the activities of physicians working in complex systems; taking care of patients over the course of their illness; and, as before, using the superior training and knowledge of physicians to advance the health of populations.

In summary, the authors describe the paradox in leading and managing healthcare professionals and also provide a direction for moving forward. Physicians and non-physician medical professionals need to be better trained in team-based communication and coordination skills. Healthcare organizations need to develop a patient-centered culture where care pathways are organized around how patients present and provide the information technology infrastructure so that the same information is available to all team members. Finally, integrated organizations need to have embedded systems that can resolve conflicts, reduce variations, monitor outcomes, recognize and reward behavior, and provide feedback loops to the care teams so they can continually improve the care process.

6

HOW HEALTH PROFESSIONAL TRAINING WILL AND SHOULD CHANGE

Alan Dow and Scott Reeves

Introduction

The demographic, economic, and quality challenges facing healthcare will require new systems of care more focused on populations, value, and collaboration. In this chapter, we explore the implications of these changes for the future healthcare workforce. Typical graduates of an educational program in the health professions have ahead of them a 30-year career during which practice will and must change dramatically. Educators, researchers, and leaders in education in the health professions must be aware of the shifting landscape. Indeed, these challenges also present an opportunity to rethink such education and to design programs that graduates entering the workforce will need to meet in an evolving healthcare system. To that end, we briefly review the history of change in education in the health professions. Then, we examine interprofessional education as a current example of change in education for health professionals as well as some other trends in modern educational practice. Finally, we outline some key principles needed to drive the educational changes for training tomorrow's healthcare workforce.

Key Moments of Change in the Education of Health Professionals

Arguably, the most transformative moment of modern education for the health professions in North America was publication of the Flexner Report in 1910 (Flexner,

1910). For this report, Abraham Flexner visited physician training sites across the United States and Canada and, based on his observations, sought to identify the approach he believed to be most beneficial to society. Flexner observed that physician training was heterogeneous and often insufficient. He advocated for significant reform of medical training. He recommended that physicians receive 4 years of undergraduate education followed by 4 years of medical school. He believed students should be trained in medical schools that were university-based with accompanying hospital affiliations, and the focus of this training should be in applying the scientific method to clinical care.

This report had profound effects on North American medical education and medicine more generally (Starr, 1982). The model outlined by Flexner has been the approach for educating physicians in the United States and many other countries for more than a century. Initially, the number of medical schools decreased from 160 to 66 as state and national medical societies increased their power over licensure and credentialing based on his ideals. Yet, because of this consolidation, medicine developed a centralized approach to education, licensure, and practice that increased the power, prestige, and wealth of physicians. The alignment of professional and educational institutions not only enhanced education but also supported the profession's rise to prominence.

The Flexner Report also had an impact on other professions. As physicians became better trained and that expertise led to increasing professional power and organization, other professions attempted to adapt similarly. The Goldmark Report (Goldmark, 1923) attempted to provide the stimulus for professionalization of nursing that the Flexner Report provided for medicine. Yet, despite a call for university-based nursing education programs, nursing education through universities remained in the minority—in part because of the larger workforce needs. The training of nursing never became aligned with traditional universities to the same degree that medical training did. The diffuse nature of nursing training is borne out today in variable approaches to education (such as tension about whether online approaches are comparable to in-person training) and competing systems for accreditation.

This contrast between medicine and nursing extends into the practice environment. While physician professional organizations such as the American Medical Association aligned with state medical societies and licensing boards to advocate for both physician autonomy and increased physician compensation, state boards of nursing took a more adversarial role toward policing the nursing profession. For medicine, the centralization of training in universities overseen by a single accreditor matched the single voice with which professional societies and licensing boards advocated for the professions. Such coordination was not evident in nursing and other professions.

However, such differences between physicians and other health professions are decreasing. In the recent Future of Nursing report (Institute of Medicine [IOM], 2011), nursing leaders outlined a new vision for increasing the professionalization and expertise of nursing. Driven by the urgency of the challenges facing the health-care system, this report outlined a consolidated approach for increasing the educational attainment of the nursing profession as a whole in order to better address the unmet needs of society and also increase the stature of the nursing profession. This vision describes the need for expanded roles of nurses at all levels of education in order to improve health. Many of these expanded roles build on increasing responsibilities for certain levels of training already in place—for example, the increasing number of master's-level nurse practitioners in primary care. The dominant theme throughout the Future of Nursing report is ensuring expertise through education and leveraging that expertise to improve health. If the medical profession is a model, these changes will also increase the stature and professional power of nursing.

Like nursing, other professions have evolved increasing bases of expertise over the past few decades. Until the 1960s, pharmacists were trained to dispense medications and specifically discouraged from counseling patients. All questions from patients were to be referred back to a physician. Over the succeeding decades, pharmacists have embraced their expertise in medications, particularly as patient needs and medications have become more complex (Sitkin & Sutcliffe, 1991). Schools of pharmacy have added curriculum on clinical assessment and patient communication, and many pharmacy students pursue pharmacy residencies to enhance their clinical abilities. Pharmacists, in some settings, prescribe and manage medications and counsel patients relatively autonomously (Emmerton, Marriott, Bessell, Nissen, & Dean, 2005). These pharmacist-led approaches have been shown to improve outcomes for patient with chronic diseases such as diabetes (Cramer, Bunting, & Christensen, 2003). Like nursing, pharmacy—perhaps the most community-embedded profession—seems poised to fill unmet health needs as the role and expertise of pharmacists expand.

Similar trends of increasing expertise can be seen across other health fields as well as these fields anticipate larger roles in primary care. For example, many programs in occupational and physical therapy now result in a professional doctorate rather than a master's degree. This additional training is seen as necessary for a more complex and evidence-based clinical world (American Occupational Therapy Association, 2014). An example of this evolution is embedding occupational or physical therapy in primary care with a focus on preventing injury rather than rehabilitating patients after they suffer injury. The overall trend is that the training of more expert professionals is leading to new and broader applications in the health system that improves the well-being of the population and increase the leadership role of these practitioners.

Yet, a more expert and diverse workforce can also increase the complexity of care. Although expertise is good for addressing a single problem, the division of labor inherent in such expertise can also lead to incoherence in the overall plan of care for a patient or population. This can create gaps where errors and inefficiencies occur.

In addition, as recommended by Flexner, training for most health professionals has been integrated into academic health centers where the greatest amount of research-driven expertise can be found. Although this approach has clear and important benefits to training experts, only one in a thousand individuals is estimated to receive care in an academic center each month (White, Williams, & Greenberg, 1961). In other words, almost all care is actually delivered outside of the educational sites in which most healthcare professionals are trained. This gap between the places where patients most often receive care and where the healthcare workforce is trained has significant implications for the future delivery of healthcare services. For example, despite the emphasis on accountable care organizations by policymakers, academic medical centers are poorly equipped to enter into these types of models (Berkowitz & Miller, 2011; Kastor, 2011). Accountable care models emphasize population-based approaches with a focus on primary care, whereas the traditional strength of academic centers is in tertiary care and specialized services. Indeed, academic centers may be further hindering the primary care transformation needed by society by not training a workforce responsive to the current changes sweeping much of the delivery system external to academic centers (Hoff, 2010).

With the healthcare system transforming, education in the health professions seems poised for change as well. A university-based model of expertise has made medicine the dominant profession of the last century. However, more recently, the needs of society have fueled changes in education in the health professions, especially outside of medicine. The changes in the population and practice portends a large impact on education. Perhaps, these professions are experiencing their own "Flexnerian moment" where expertise, responsiveness to community needs, and bridging gaps between experts will redefine health education and the health services delivered to society.

Driver of Change: The Intersection of Education and Practice

In a report on the global healthcare workforce earlier this decade, Frenk et al. (2010) described the current separation between education in the health professions and healthcare delivery. The report noted students are usually trained at institutions of higher education that either are removed from the delivery of healthcare or deliver healthcare in a subsidized fashion atypical of usual practice. At the same time, healthcare delivery organizations provide most of their care without the involvement of learners (or researchers) on whom the future of the organization depends. Many of the challenges facing healthcare delivery may have roots in this separation.

Yet, the links between these two sectors are many. Clearly, graduates of educational programs in health professions become the workforce of healthcare organizations. Less obvious, but perhaps more important, is that students, faculty, and staff are also consumers of the health services provided by trainees of educational programs. Learners, for example, may have experiences as patients or family members of patients within the healthcare system. These experiences shape their professional identities and their vision for the kind of healthcare system in which they wish to practice and receive their own services. Faculty and staff from educational institutions are likewise influenced by their experiences as consumers of health services. As such, the Frenk report asserted that education and practice should be viewed as part of the same ecosystem. The report advocates that, given the health challenges facing society, acknowledging and strengthening these relationships may be essential to transform health education and health services delivery.

In the United States, there is some evidence that the gap between education and practice has begun to narrow. Clinical service constituted only 6% of medical school revenues in 1961 but 52% of medical school revenues in 2008 (Miller et al., 2012). As tuition shrank from 6% to 3% of revenues and federal research funding fell from 31% to 19% over these four decades, medical schools became much more focused on healthcare delivery and much less reliant on other revenue sources such as tuition. Medical schools have responded by becoming less focused on education and research and more focused on clinical practice. Likewise, institutions that educate nursing and other health professionals have seen a closer alignment between practice and education. Many nonacademic health systems have begun their own schools for training and maintaining a workforce pipeline. In addition, the proliferation of online programs has allowed students to work and train concurrently and move up the ranks of the organization and profession. Individuals who progress from certified nursing assistants to licensed practical nurses to registered nurses to bachelor's-prepared registered nurses, all while working as part of the nursing team full-time, are common examples. These opportunities benefit both individuals—who can grow into a more rewarding career—and systems that reap the benefit of well-trained and loyal employees.

But in spite of the narrowing gap between education and practice, new entrants into the healthcare workforce appear to lack some of the abilities needed to thrive in the current system or drive the change needed for an improved system (IOM, 2003).

Despite the ideal of healthy communities, education tends to focus on individuals rather than populations and episodic care rather than ongoing health. In addition, healthcare is delivered increasingly by interprofessional teams, yet interprofessional education remains a developing field and many of teams in healthcare function suboptimally (IOM, 2015). And, although evidence-based practice had matured into an integrated part of most curricula, innovations with proven benefit still takes too long to be applied in practice.

Shortfalls such as these have engendered a discussion about the meaning of professional competence (Epstein & Hundert, 2002) and a movement in health professions education toward competency-based education (Holmboe, Sherbino, Long, Swing, & Frank, 2010). Under a model of competency-based education, instruction and assessment in a curriculum is driven by competencies—the defined abilities a practicing professional must have to function effectively in a role. For example, all healthcare practitioners need the competency of being able to collaborate effectively with other health professions to meet the needs of patients, families, and communities. This competency should then drive instruction and assessment around collaboration and teamwork.

The emphasis on defining and educating to competence is perhaps the strongest current in health professions education at present. It signifies the desire of educators to graduate a workforce more prepared to meet the needs of society rather than an internal standard of expertise. It also captures the struggle of defining the necessary professional abilities for a practitioner in an evolving healthcare environment and developing curriculum that ensures that the practitioner has these abilities.

Interprofessional Education as a Case Study of Change in Health Professions Education

Describing the needs for improved teamwork in healthcare, the World Health Organization (2010) defined collaborative practice as "when multiple health workers from different professional backgrounds provide comprehensive services by working with patients, their families, careers and communities to deliver the highest quality of care across settings" (p. 13). Furthermore, this report described interprofessional education as "when two or more professions learn about, from, and with each other to enable effective collaboration and improve health outcomes" (p. 13). Three features of this definition for interprofessional education are notable.

First, it specifies two challenging goals for educators: enabling collaboration and improving health outcomes. Enabling collaboration is challenging because of the traditional divides between academic programs. However, improving health outcomes—presumably the goal of all activities in health professions education—is even more challenging. Although we can use process measures of learning activities to assess the question of whether interprofessional education enables collaboration, it is more difficult to demonstrate the effect of any educational change on outcomes. In fact, the number of interprofessional education interventions that have been demonstrated to improve health outcomes is small (IOM, 2015). Although this number has been increasing (Reeves et al., 2008; Reeves, Perrier, Goldman, Freeth, & Zwarenstein, 2013), implementing effective interprofessional education as measured by an impact on health outcomes remains largely aspirational. Despite this shortcoming, however, the definition of interprofessional education places this approach squarely at the intersection of education and practice.

Second, it reports that the prepositions "about, from, and with" in the definition of interprofessional education imply students not just learning together but also teaching or facilitating the learning from each other. This colearning approach has become increasingly emphasized in health education of single professions through approaches such as problem-based learning (Albanese & Mitchell, 1993). Problem-based learning replaces traditional lecture with small group interaction that emphasizes collaboration around learning materials. A problem-based approach seems to improve learning, especially retention of concepts, and it is also resource-intensive because a higher faculty-to-student ratio is needed to support collaborative activities by students. Interprofessional education faces similar challenges. Indeed, interprofessional education is resource-intensive, and the cost of programs is a significant barrier (Lawlis, Anson, & Greenfield, 2014). Yet, positioning learners as teachers relative to their peers from other professions is essential for developing teams where shared expertise can be valued and flourish.

Finally, although this definition had been evolving for decades, it was only widely accepted in 2010. Although educators in the health professions have been advocating interprofessional education for decades (IOM, 1972), this concept of educating to increase teamwork in healthcare has been very slow to take hold. The publication of the "To Err is Human" report (IOM, 1999) identified inadequate teamwork as a major cause of the thousands of preventable deaths that occur each year in the United States. Additional research has continually shown that poor communication and leadership are implicated as a cause of approximately two thirds of sentinel events reported to the Joint Commission (The Joint Commission, 2014). These findings led the Institute of Medicine (IOM) to call for interprofessional education as one of five important areas of focus for health professions education (IOM, 2003). Over the next 10 years, that recommendation has translated into accrediting standards for all of the largest health fields requiring interprofessional education (Zorek & Raehl, 2013). This initiative has been furthered by the Liaison Committee on

Medical Education, the accreditor for medical schools, beginning to require medical schools to have interprofessional activities in the summer of 2014. Despite a slow start, over the past decade interprofessional education has become a priority for education in the health professions.

Yet, hidden in this progress around accreditation standards remains an example of the challenges going forward: each profession has a profession-specific standard for interprofessional education. Certain professions are more explicit in their accreditation standards about the criteria for interprofessional education (such as pharmacy and dentistry), whereas other professions (such as nursing) have accrediting standards that are less prescriptive. Although a common accrediting standard has been suggested as a need in the future, it is unclear how that might evolve and be applied. For example, professions that graduate greater numbers of professionals each year (such as nursing) have a much more difficult time finding partners for interprofessional education.

Indeed, despite a widely accepted definition and the adoption of accrediting standards, many challenges remain to implementing interprofessional education. The best methods for instruction and assessment are still being defined. For example, some institutions have developed classroom-based courses, whereas others have created simulation-based experiences. Practice-based experiences intuitively seem the most promising, yet these experiences are the most costly, and most systems struggle to provide clinical settings that embody effective interprofessional practice. Likely, the best approaches for interprofessional education will be costly to develop and maintain, and determining the cost-effectiveness of interprofessional education may be a challenge faced by educators and leaders in this area. Perhaps the evolution of the healthcare delivery system may provide some new opportunities about which educators can capitalize to close the education–practice gap and train more interprofessional practitioners.

The most pressing concern related to interprofessional education is how to implement continuing education and workplace training. Most of the innovation in interprofessional education has occurred in degree programs, yet the urgency of the changing healthcare system suggests the need for workforce evolution is already upon us. What, then, should be done about continuing professional development? Should current practitioners have interprofessional education requirements as part of their ongoing certification process? Overall, continuing education generally has limited evidence of its effectiveness on practice outcomes (Bordage, Carlin, Mazmanian, & American College of Chest Physicians Health and Science Policy Committee, 2009), and this extends to when continuing education is used to deliver interprofessional content specifically (Evans, Mazmanian, Dow, Lockeman, & Yanchick, 2014). Because educators for both continuing education and interprofessional education are anxious to develop programs with more demonstrated impact on practice, integrating interprofessional learning into continuing education might represent an approach for better representing the complexity of practice and increasing the impact of continuing education (Owens & Schmitt, 2013). Although the motivation to increase interprofessional education is established, how to implement instruction and assessment with impact are questions that continue to drive the field.

An Example of Evidence of Effectiveness: Team Training to Reduce Errors

The approach to interprofessional education most supported by the evidence is team training—education that focuses on enhancing collaboration within existing, discrete clinical teams. On the heels of the IOM reports linking poor communication among healthcare practitioners and harmful errors (IOM, 1999, 2001), healthcare leaders and educators became interested in the concept of team training for healthcare practitioners. Team training in nonhealthcare fields has been demonstrated to enhance team performance (Salas et al., 2008). As a result, these nonhealthcare concepts for team training have been translated to healthcare settings through several programs, most notably the TeamSTEPPS program funded by the Agency for Healthcare Research and Quality (Baker, Gustafson, Beaubien, Salas, & Barach, 2005). This freely available program provides training and assessment methods for educators, including an overarching training framework and specific lessons across a variety of clinical settings (King et al., 2008). A similar team training approach, crew resource management, has also been adopted from outside healthcare. These approaches seem to be linked to clinical benefits (Neily, et al. 2010, 2011; Salas, Gregory, & King, 2011), although the effect of a training intervention in a complex healthcare system has multiple possible confounders.

However, these approaches have not been widely integrated for reasons inherent to the training and delivery of healthcare. The evidence supports team training but also says these teams must have discretely defined membership (Salas et al., 2008). Although team training works, when new individuals join the team or existing members leave the team, the benefits are attenuated. Healthcare, in particular, has fluid and poorly defined teams (Reeves, Lewin, Espin, & Zwarenstein, 2010), and team training lessons may not lead to gains that translate from one team to the next.

Consider the following example. Supposing an inpatient nurse is caring for four patients, each of whom is cared for by four medical (physician) teams. Thus, the nurse could be considered part of four teams. As time moves forward, say the following day, that nurse may be off duty. Now, the four patients assigned to that nurse the previous day may be assigned to one to four new nurses, creating four new teams caring for these four patients. Meanwhile, patients may leave the hospital, and new patients are admitted, transitioning between outpatient and inpatient teams. That nurse who returns to work from being off duty may have four new patients with four new medical teams. Also, the care of each of these patients is governed by different relationships between the healthcare workers, the system, and the patient.

As such, healthcare teams are often not discrete, intact entities, focused on a single product such work teams in many other industries. The successful studies of team training in healthcare have focused primarily on more discrete teams with stable membership, such as surgical teams (Neily et al., 2010, 2011). How to develop generalizable teamwork competency is less clear. Indeed, given the fluidity of interprofessional practice in healthcare, arguably we ought to be thinking about developing competency approaches that more realistically reflect these shifting patterns of practice—from coordination, networking, and collaboration (Reeves et al., 2010). With the bulk of health professions education occurring in the prelicensure phase rather than in the workplace, this question is especially imperative under the current model for health professions education.

Defining Goals for Interprofessional Education

If education in the health professions should focus on developing generalizable collaborative competencies at the prelicensure level, then educators need to consider proxy measures for evaluating the effectiveness of educational programs that link to ideal interprofessional practice. Unfortunately, as previously noted, interprofessional practice itself is poorly defined (Goldman, Zwarenstein, Bhattacharyya, & Reeves, 2009). Although teamwork in nonhealthcare settings has developed an evidence base to shape evaluation and training (Morgeson, DeRue, & Karam, 2010), only a few of these concepts have been brought over to healthcare (Dow, DiazGranados, Mazmanian, & Retchin, 2013). A greater understanding of effective interprofessional work is essential to identify the interprofessional education interventions that lead to better interprofessional practice.

A key acclaimed event for shaping interprofessional education in the United States was the publication of the Core Competencies for Interprofessional Collaborative Practice (Interprofessional Education Collaborative Expert Panel, 2011). Developed by twelve leaders from six health professions, the competencies were designed to serve as standards for graduating students for health professions programs. They consist of four domains: values and ethics, roles and responsibilities, interprofessional communication, and teams and teamwork. The competencies have shaped the dialogue around interprofessional education and have shown some promise for describing and measuring interprofessional competency (Dow, DiazGranados, Mazmanian, & Retchin, 2014). Yet, many educators have found the competencies challenging to apply to specific educational experiences and also have found difficulties with robustly assessing these competencies (Reeves, 2012). As a next step, the field needs to move beyond expert opinion and toward truly evidence-based understanding of the competencies that support effective interprofessional practice.

The lack of consensus about goals for interprofessional education manifests itself in the published literature in interprofessional education. The educational approaches are heterogeneous, and most reported outcomes are short-term (Abu-Rish et al., 2012). In addition, the program evaluations are dissimilar such that comparisons between programs or analyses of collective outcomes are unmanageable. Educators and researchers need better frameworks to guide the development, implementation, evaluation, and assessment of interprofessional education so that a true benefit can be ensured.

Other Changing Trends in Education in the Health Professions

ADMITTING THE RIGHT INDIVIDUALS FOR THE HEALTHCARE WORKFORCE OF THE FUTURE

As educators and policymakers have identified the need for a differently trained healthcare workforce, they have begun to look at the admissions process to educational programs in the health professions. Admission to nearly all educational programs in the health professions is competitive, and, as such, programs have the opportunity to be selective about the individuals they admit. The opportunity for selectivity is being leveraged in innovative ways.

The most marked change in the admitting process is the revision of the Medical College Admissions Test (MCAT) in 2015. The revised test focuses more on the humanistic aspects of medicine such as how illness and disease interact with society broadly (Dienstag, 2011). Content such as ethics, population health, and culture have been given increased emphasis. In addition, the test authors seek to have examinees apply scientific knowledge within more complex context through critical thinking and reasoning. In a sense then, the revised MCAT is also seeking to bridge the gap between science-based education and the evolving practice needs of society. How the test succeeds at identifying a more optimal future workforce will be an issue of interest over the next decade.

Some institutions are also taking specific steps to improve the admissions process. The multiple mini-interview is one innovation in the admissions process that has gained traction in a number of medical schools (Eva, Rosenfeld, Reiter, & Norman, 2004). An applicant to a typical medical school has one interview, lasting about an hour, with a faculty member. This interview is critical to the admissions decision and relies on the judgment of the faculty member about the applicant. Yet this judgment has been found to be problematic, both in its accuracy and reproducibility (Harasym, Woloschuk, Mandin, & Brundin-Mather, 1996). To overcome the limitation of having a single rater of each applicant, the mini-interview was introduced. In the mini-interview, an applicant interacts with about a dozen faculty members across a number of short interactions. Each faculty member has a specific focus and compares a succession of applicants across a short period. The faculty member can more accurately assess each applicant in comparison to the broader applicant pool and in the specific areas of focus defined by the school. This approach has been shown to correlate with scores on licensing examinations (Eva et al., 2012) and practice-based assessments (Eva et al., 2009) later in medical school. As mini-interviews are adopted by other schools and health professions, the impact of this approach on the healthcare workforce overall will be another to track.

SIMULATION-BASED EDUCATION

In addition to interprofessional education, other approaches to education in the health professions are helping to frame the future of training the healthcare workforce. Simulation-based education has become a high-profile method for instruction and assessment in such education over the past 15 years. As a more mature instructional approach than interprofessional education, the debate around simulation-based education is more crystallized around defining educational value (Brydges, Hatala, Zendejas, Erwin, & Cook, 2015). Defined broadly, simulation-based education involves replicating any aspect of the clinical environment to support learning. Although much of simulation-based education relies on technology such as high-fidelity simulators, simulation-based education can also include the use of standardized patients (i.e., actors portraying fictional patients), computer-based education, and lower fidelity simulators such as teaching laparoscopic surgical skills using box trainers (i.e., hollow cubes that obstruct the operator's line of sight so that the operator must rely on his or her tactile input and the laparoscopic camera to perform operative techniques). Each of these categories is important for educators trying to select the best educational approach (Hammoud et al., 2008).

The rise in importance of simulation-based education over the past two decades stems from several sources. First, the technology available for simulation-based education has flourished as computing has advanced. Simulators have become much better at representing clinical situations (the concept of fidelity) while also much easier for educators to program and operate. Costs for a specific simulator have also decreased.

Second, the emphasis on competency-based education (Holmboe et al., 2010) has attuned educators to the need to assess specific aspects of clinical performance more carefully. Perhaps the best example of this trend is the adoption of the US Medical Licensing Examination, or USMLE, Step 2 clinical skills examination during which medical students are scored by standardized patients on their communication skills. Passage is required to enter clinical practice. Defining specific areas of competency—in this example, physician–patient communication—has led to the creation of new assessment approaches that are not only applied by licensing organizations but also in programs of study as they train students for that assessment modality.

The third, and perhaps most important, reason for the growth of simulation-based education is the movement of clinical teaching away from the bedside. Over the past decades, the Flexnerian ideal of patient-centered clinical education has been challenged by the need to ensure the safety of patients and minimize the medicolegal risk of teaching hospitals. In the past, students would learn to perform procedures on patients under the mantra of "see one, do one, teach one"—a student's first attempt at phlebotomy or a spinal tap would be on a real patient. To better protect patients and limit their discomfort, simulation-based education has been introduced into training. Instead of students learning initially with patients, they show competence in simulation prior to performing the actual procedure on a patient.

Well-designed simulation-based education can be effective, but the instructional approach matters (McGaghie, Issenberg, Barsuk, & Wayne, 2014). For example, the instructional approach with the best-studied results is directed practice. During directed practice, a student is supervised by an instructor while repeatedly performing a learning task. The student receives ongoing feedback from the simulator or instructor and progresses to the next segment of learning (usually a more difficult task or subsequent step of the task) after demonstrating mastery of the previous task. Directed practice has been shown to be superior to other approaches for in situ learning in simulation, including benefits for transference of simulation-based learning to the clinical environment and an impact on clinical outcomes.

Yet, directed practice is a task-based approach that may have less relevance for some of the challenges facing health education. Although directed practice is useful for technical expertise, how this model can be applied to areas such as interprofessional interactions and the complexity of team-based care is unclear. Whether repeated coaching around learning focused on human interaction can improve workplace performance is unknown. Simulation-based education clearly meets an educational need in health professions, and now the limits of its applicability need to be defined.

Simulation-based education has also uncovered some important learning principles that may be widely applicable in education in the health professions. Despite a focus on technology, how well a simulator models real life may be less important than assumed by many (Curtis & Feldman, 2012; Norman, Dore, & Grierson, 2012). High-fidelity simulators that more closely mimic the clinical environment may be worse for learning in certain situations. For example, providing a novice learner with a high-fidelity experience can distract from the core learning goals by overloading the learners with information. This "cognitive overload" can lead to worse learning outcomes. In essence, as evidence by directed practice, the key to simulation-based education is understanding the learning goals of an educational experience and titrating the context and feedback within the training to the desired outcomes (Hamstra, Brydges, Hatala, Zendejas, & Cook, 2014). Sometimes, less is more—a tenet that may have value for other approaches in health professions education.

Simulation-based education should continue to expand. Despite its demonstrated effectiveness, simulation-based education is still unevenly and inadequately adopted into educational practice (McGaghie et al., 2014). The ideal of certifying competence in simulation prior to performing a procedure on a patient has not been achieved. Perhaps the biggest barrier to simulation-based education is cost. Simulation-based education often requires expensive equipment and a greater investment of faculty time than other instructional methods, yet research on simulation-based education rarely reports data on cost (Zanedjas, Wang, Brydges, Hamstra, & Cook, 2013). Much of the slow expansion of simulation-based education likely stems from the uncertainty of how to balance the benefits of simulation-based education with the costs of implementing a more expensive instructional approach. Where a ready funding source is apparent, simulation-based education has grown. For example, the board of anesthesiology requires simulation-based education for recertification of anesthesiologists and requires the recertifying anesthesiologists to pay for these assessments. Recertifying anesthesiologists as practitioners who must manage infrequent but life-threatening complications through simulation-based education makes sense for training these professionals, and the fees paid by the recertifying practitioners provides a reliable funding source.

Yet, many other arenas in health education lack the impetus for significant integration of simulation-based education. For example, although training residents to insert central lines with simulation is superior for learning and patient outcomes (Khouli et al., 2011), this approach is not required across healthcare. Successful integration of an educational change will require evidence of value and cohesive leadership to advocate for these best practices. Meanwhile, although simulation-based education is a mature approach for task-based learning, it has only begun to be studied and adopted for more complex learning areas such as interprofessional education (Fung et al., 2015). From dissemination across professions to application for new approaches, simulation-based education promises to continue to evolve.

LONGITUDINAL INTEGRATED CLERKSHIPS

Another trend in health education is the introduction of longitudinal integrated clerkships for medical students. Traditionally, third-year medical students spend 4 to 12 weeks in a variety of medical specialties such as surgery, pediatrics, and internal medicine. This rotation exposes students to different medical specialties while also providing them opportunities to consider each specialty as a career. However, some educators believe this approach needs to be reexamined. Because clinical practice varies so much by specialty, transitioning among specialties means students have to learn the practical aspects of care for each venue every few weeks. In addition, this approach discourages continuity and has been blamed for the decreasing number of primary care-oriented medical school graduates. Consequently, a few medical schools in the United States and elsewhere have adopted longitudinal integrated clerkships (Norris et al., 2009). In this model, students have an ongoing experience with a panel of patients that spans a longer period of time, usually an academic year. Students have more continuity with patients, faculty, and clinical sites.

Students in longitudinal integrated clerkships appear to have better clinical skills and equivalent medical knowledge to students in transitional models (Walters et al., 2012; Teherani, Irby, & Loeser, 2013). These outcomes seem to stem from students having closer relationships with faculty from whom they receive more feedback on performance. However, it is not clear that any benefits from this educational approach extend into residency (Woloschuk, Myhre, Jackson, McLaughlin, & Wright, 2014). Like other novel educational approaches in the health professions, the desired benefits have a sound theoretical basis, but demonstrating efficacy over the long term is problematic and confounded by many other factors.

However, longitudinal integrated clerkships are notable for two reasons. First, they represent a recent example of the willingness of medical education to change to address some of the issues facing medicine, in particular declines in empathy among students, lack of interest in primary care, and a disconnect between faculty and students. As a challenge to the Flexnerian model, they are emblematic of the desire of medical education to evolve. Second, a longitudinal model for clinical training where one or more students are paired with a preceptor for a semester is typical of education in nursing and other health professional programs. Perhaps after 100 years, medicine is realizing a shortcoming of the Flexnerian approach and a strength of other areas of health professions education.

THE LENGTH AND VALUE OF TRAINING

Another trend in the education of health professionals is reconsidering the length of training or segments of training. In nursing and other fields, many programs are increasing the length of training. As noted, physical therapy and occupational therapy programs are moving from a master's degree as the practice-entry degree to a doctoral degree. These changes add an additional one to three semesters to training, which, to date, seems acceptable to applicants. Similarly, nursing education has evolved because of evidence suggesting a relationship between nurses' educational level and quality of patient care. The most prominent recent study demonstrated that, for each 10% increase in the number of nurses with a bachelor's degree at a hospital, the 30-day hospital mortality decreased 7% (Aiken et al., 2014). Findings such as this have led to goals such as increasing the number of nurses with a bachelors from 50% to 80% (IOM, 2011). Institutions that train nurses also have numerous programs to add credentials, ranging from master's degrees and practice doctoral degrees to specialty certifications. At the root of all of these changes is expanded expertise through longer training with a focus on evidence-based practice, leadership, quality improvement, and interprofessional collaboration.

Yet in medicine, the trend is the opposite. The Flexnerian approach of having two preclinical years was in favor for more than 100 years, but most medical schools are now shifting to preclinical training that lasts 18 months or less. Medical educators seem motivated by a desire to increase the length of clinical training of their students. However, the fourth year of medical school—the portion extended by most recent curricular reforms—is the least structured part of medical education (Wolf, Lockspeiser, Gong, & Guiton, 2014), and its utility has long been questioned. In fact, some medical schools have begun to graduate students in 3 years. Because the largest barrier to earlier graduation from medical school is the need for graduating medical students to participate in the residency match, programs that graduate students in 3 years link entry into the program with placement in an affiliated family medicine residency. By design, these programs seek to increase the quantity of the students entering primary care. As a result, we may see an occupational therapist in primary care whose schooling lasted as long as medical school.

Why is education in medicine different from that in the other health professions in this regard? With fewer medical students entering primary care (Jeffe, Whelan, & Andriole, 2010), these accelerated programs are designed to increase the number of students choosing primary care. Yet it is unclear that the economic benefits of simply "lopping off" a year of medical school will promote such a shift in interest, and because the existing programs ask students to commit to the track during their first year, most of the graduates enter medical school oriented toward primary care and remain as such through graduation. Still, the changes in the training duration for medicine and other professions have a similar impetus: the desire to better meet the needs for society.

What the approach of medicine to these needs will mean for medical education overall remains to be seen. Scientific knowledge continues to expand, and medical students are asked to master this information in a shorter period of time. Medical schools then look to antecedent education to better prepare students in the sciences while admission processes (and society) are looking for more well-rounded students. This paradox is challenging for potential applicants and may erode the scientific foundation of future physicians. At the same time, medical schools are implementing new instructional techniques to make learning more efficient. For example, in the "flipped classroom," students receive lectures outside of the classroom over the Internet and use class time to discuss and apply the lecture material. This model is based on learning theory and evidence, but its effectiveness varies depending on the instructor, the content, and other factors (Khanova, Roth, Rodgers, & McLaughlin, 2015). Faced with increasing pressures to do more with less, medical education needs evidence to define the efficacy and applicability of various approaches, particularly because other health professions have chosen to extend rather than shorten training. These outcomes must be evaluated with a long time horizon.

Driving all of health education should be the question of how it impacts patient and community outcomes. The cost of education continues to increase substantially, whether from lengthening training for nonphysicians or the rising cost for similar durations of training in medical school (Greysen, Chen, & Mullan, 2011). These costs have implications for workforce development, ranging from decisions on matriculation to career choice such as entering primary care. Without evidence of educational efficacy to patients and communities, an educational program's value—benefit divided by cost—is strictly a financial calculation at the level of the individual student in terms of that individual's salary and lifestyle preferences. To optimize the healthcare workforce, we need to understand the benefit of training different kinds of professionals in different ways so that we can allocate resources to the most valuable programs in our society (Walsh, 2015).

Implications for Practice, Theory, and Research

Given the changes in the US health care system, the implications for the education of health professionals are enormous. Because today's trainees are the workforce of the next several decades, how people are trained today shapes the care generations of people will receive. It is this realization that spurs the need to bring education, practice, and communities closer together (Frenk et al., 2010). Although concerns about clinical errors initiated this direction (IOM, 2001), all of education needs to be evaluated within the framework of not just safety but also how it addresses the health needs of populations, including access to care, cost of care, and disparities within care. A few key tenets should structure this movement going forward.

THE NEED FOR EVIDENCE OF IMPACT

Research on health professions education has been slow to mature. Flexner's original report was a descriptive survey of a number of medical schools that drew conclusions based on his assessment of the quality of the graduating physician workforce. These conclusions shaped a century of education of health professionals.

Today, our understanding of the impact of different education programs in the health professions is arguably only slightly better. Curricular decisions often rely more on expert opinion than evidence. Expanding and adding rigor to educational research on health professions education are critical as we enter a time of great change in preparation of the healthcare workforce.

There is reason to be optimistic about research in education in the health professions. The number of educators trained as researchers is increasing. An increasing number of conferences and journals focused on educational research support this trend in the health professions. Meanwhile, scientists, particularly social scientists, are increasingly bringing their expertise to bear on the challenges of educating the health workforce in a highly effective manner. The various educational interventions discussed in this chapter are examples of how scientists from inside and outside the health professions have shaped interventions by adding rigor and creativity to the evaluation of innovations in education of health professionals.

Yet the main question remains as to what curricular interventions have an impact on the practicing healthcare workforce and, most importantly, the health of the population. Perhaps the single greatest barrier to demonstrating the impact of different approaches to education in the health professions is tracking learners as they diffuse into practice and begin to affect communities. This area is fraught with challenges—studying heterogeneous communities served by networks of healthcare practitioners is complex—but, as a starting point, a registry of graduating healthcare practitioners that links metrics of academic performance, certification and licensing information, clinical data, and patient outcomes could support evaluating the impact of education on healthcare practice. Such ambitious thinking is necessary if we are to truly understand the innovations that really matter in education of health professionals.

DEFINING AND DEMONSTRATING COMPETENCY

If a set of abilities or competencies is necessary to practice in a health profession, these abilities should be discretely defined. Trainees and practitioners should demonstrate these competencies prior to practice and be assessed for maintenance of competency. Competencies necessarily evolve as science advances, and practitioners will need retraining.

In some areas of clinical practice, such as simulation-based education for central line placement, the competencies are well-defined and effective training models exist. Accreditors, licensing bodies, and other organizations with professional authority should exert their power here to benefit patients. In other areas, such as interprofessional practice, competencies are less well defined. Educators and researchers should work with practitioners to define practical and valid competency frameworks. These frameworks can then be applied to curricula across the educational spectrum from novices to practitioners seeking continuing education.

Demonstrating competency also has implications for research on the overall impact of health professions education outlined above. If competencies can be used as clear criteria of performance, the impact of achieving competency at an individual, organizational, or community level can be linked to population health outcomes. In an ideal world, these competency assessments would follow the practitioner through formal education and into continuing education, driving training across a career. Linking these criteria to a research database could add further granularity to understanding of the impact of education in the health professions on outcomes and which approaches have the most merit.

DETERMINATION AND DISSEMINATION OF BEST MODELS

If competency is to be a guiding principle in health education, then identifying how best to train to competency is critical. Much of educational research focuses on assessing an innovation without a comparison group. As a result, leaders and educators often struggle to determine if an innovation is better or just different. To address this issue, educators and researchers should strive to develop comparative studies rather than just program descriptions. Comparisons should not be limited to short educational interventions but applied to broader questions such as what is the optimum length of undergraduate training for different health professions. Although in many instances several educational approaches may be suitable and the best approach may be shaped by contextual factors, a broad and coordinated focus on research and dissemination is essential to develop evidence around different educational approaches and to have a positive impact on health outcomes. As above, coordination between educational and practice entities and a database of outcomes are essential for moving this dialogue forward.

TRAINING FOR LIFELONG LEARNING

Patient-centered educational outcomes must consider both current and future patients. Essential to improving the health of future patients is training health professionals to be "master learners"—individuals with the ability and desire to continually improve their practice (Schumacher, Englander, & Carraccio, 2013). Training master learners requires cultivating an intrinsic motivation for learning in individuals while also equipping them with the capacity to accurately self-assess learning needs and access appropriate continuing education. In a changing world, these abilities are critical. Education in the health professions has begun to adopt these concepts with competency domains such as "self-directed learning" or "practice-based improvement."

To further support this ideal, continuing education reform is essential. The IOM has called for continuing education to be more practice-focused, including a greater interprofessional emphasis (IOM, 2009). The next step in this evolution is moving away from hour-based credit and toward outcome-based or competency-based credit that rewards continuing education that changes how care is delivered. This redesign will require planners and faculty to approach continuing education differently. Rather than the typical lecture developed and presented by a clinical expert, education will need to focus on practitioner-defined needs and training to develop practice-centered interventions that seek to engage patients and improve health outcomes.

UNDERSTANDING COST AND VALUE

Education in the health professions has often been insulated from cost. Although tuition dollars drive much of the funding of this education, students have proven to be relatively cost-insensitive. For example, during the Great Recession, law schools saw tremendous declines in enrollment while health professional training programs actually saw increases in applicants. Yet costs can no longer be ignored, both in practice and education. The cost of medical education is blamed for the decreasing interest in primary care of medical students and spurred the development of 3-year degrees for students interested in family medicine. As other professions lengthen training, costs may play a role in student choices as well.

But the real reason to understand costs in education is to determine the value of educational programs to society overall. Whether it is the length of prelicensure training, added fees for simulation-based education, or registration for continuing professional development, underlying each of these approaches is a monetary investment for which learners and society should expect a proportional benefit. In addition to defining effective models, we need to determine the cost of each approach so we can support educational interventions that have value. If a database of educational approaches, practice data, and patient outcomes is developed, cost should be a key component so that the value of health professions education can be clearly defined.

COHESIVE LEADERSHIP

To advance any of these ideas will require cohesive leadership across different segments of the health professions and society. Certainly, different groups of health professionals will need to collaborate to support interprofessional education and this work has begun. But, even bigger benefits can be reaped from collaboration among educators, practitioners, insurers, accreditors, and community members. Educators have shown a willingness to be responsive to external trends, yet they alone cannot set a course for the innovation we need in the training of the healthcare workforce. Rather, practitioners, accreditors, and insurers need to work with educators to define competency, disseminate effective programs, and reward high-performing trainees and institutions. And these efforts must include the community that is served to ensure impact on society. Although the path forward remains uncertain, only through collaboration can we train the workforce needed to optimize the health of our communities.

References

Abu-Rish, E., Kim, S., Choe, L., Varpio, L., Malik, E., White, A., . . . Zierler, B. (2012). Current trends in interprofessional education of health sciences students: A literature review. *Journal of Interprofessional Care, 26*(6), 444–451.

Aiken, L., Sloane, D., Bruyneel, L., Van den Heede, K., Griffiths, P., Busse, R., . . . Sermeus, W. (2014). Nurse staffing and education and hospital mortality in nine European countries: A retrospective observational study. *Lancet, 383*(9931), 1824–1830.

Albanese, M., & Mitchell, S. (1993). Problem-based learning: A review of literature on its outcomes and implementation issues. *Academic Medicine, 68*(1), 52–81.

American Occupational Therapy Association. (April 30, 2014). *AOTA board of directors position statement on entry-level degree for the occupational therapist.* Retrieved from American Occupational Therapy Association: http://www.aota.org/aboutaota/get-involved/bod/otd-statement.aspx

Baker, D., Gustafson, S., Beaubien, J., Salas, E., & Barach, P. (2005). *Medical teamwork and patient safety: the evidence-based relation.* Rockville, MD: Agency for Healthcare Research and Quality.

Berkowitz, S., & Miller, E. (2011). Accountable care at academic medical centers—Lessons from Johns Hopkins. *New England Journal of Medicine, 364*(7), e12.

Bordage, G., Carlin, B., Mazmanian, P., & American College of Chest Physicians Health and Science Policy Committee. (2009). Continuing medical education effect on physician knowledge: Effectiveness of continuing medical education: American College of Chest Physicians Evidence-Based Educational Guidelines. *Chest, 135,* 29S–36S.

Brydges, R., Hatala, R., Zendejas, B., Erwin, P., & Cook, D. (2015). Linking simulation-based educational assessments and patient-related outcomes: A systematic review and meta-analysis. *Academic Medicine, 90*(2), 246–256.

Cramer, C., Bunting, B., & Christensen, D. (2003). The Asheville Project: Long-term clinical and economic outcomes of a community pharmacy diabetes care program. *Journal of the American Pharmaceutical Association, 43,* 173–184.

Curtis, M. D. D., & Feldman, M. (2012). Judicious use of simulation technology in continuing medical education. *Journal of Continuing Education in the Health Professions, 32*(4), 255–260.

Dienstag, J. (2011). The medical college admission test—Toward a new balance. *New England Journal of Medicine, 365,* 1955–1957.

Dow, A., DiazGranados, D., Mazmanian, P., & Retchin, S. (2013). Applying organizational science to health care: A framework for collaborative practice. *Academic Medicine, 88*(7), 952–977.

Dow, A., DiazGranados, D., Mazmanian, P., & Retchin, S. (2014). An exploratory study of an assessment tool derived from the competencies of the interprofessional education collaborative. *Journal of Interprofessional Care, 28*(4), 299–304.

Emmerton, L., Marriott, J., Bessell, T., Nissen, L., & Dean, L. (2005). Pharmacists and prescribing rights: Review of international developments. *Journal of Pharmacy and Pharmaceutical Sciences, 8*(2), 215–225.

Epstein, R., & Hundert, E. (2002). Defining and assessing professional competence. *Journal of the American Medical Association, 287*(2), 226–235.

Eva, K., Reiter, H., Rosenfield, J., Trinh, K., Wood, T., & Norman, G. (2012). Association between a medical school admission process using the multiple mini-interview and national licensing examination scores. *Journal of the American Medical Association, 308*(21), 2233–2240.

Eva, K., Reiter, H., Trinh, K., Wasi, P., Rosenfeld, J., & Norman, G. (2009). Predictive validity of the multiple mini-interview for selecting medical trainees. *Medical Education, 43*(8), 767–775.

Eva, K., Rosenfeld, J., Reiter, H., & Norman, G. (2004). An admissions OSCE: The multiple mini-interview. *Medical Education, 38*(3), 314–326.

Evans, J., Mazmanian, P., Dow, A., Lockeman, K., & Yanchick, V. (2014). Commitment to change and assessment of confidence: Tools to inform the design and evaluation of interprofessional education. *Journal of Continuing Education in the Health Professions, 34*(3), 155–163.

Flexner, A. (1910). *Medical Education in the United States and Canada.* New York, NY: Carnegie Foundation.

Frenk, J., Chen, L., Bhutta, Z., Cohen, J., Crisp, N., Evans, T., . . . Zurayk, H. (2010). Health professionals for a new century: transforming education to strengthen health systems in an interdependent world. *Lancet, 376*(9756), 1923–1958.

Fung, L., Boet, S., Bould, M., Qosa, H., Perrier, L., Tricco, A., . . . Reeves, S. (2015). Impact of crisis resource management simulation-based training for interprofessional and interdisciplinary teams: A systematic review. *Journal of Interprofessional Care, 29*(5), 1–12.

Goldman, J., Zwarenstein, M., Bhattacharyya, O., & Reeves, S. (2009). Improving the clarity of the interprofessional field: Implications for research and continuing interprofessional education. *Journal of Continuing Education in the Health Professions, 29*(3), 151–156.

Goldmark, J. (1923). *Nursing and nursing education in the United States: Report of the committee for the study of nursing education.* New York, NY: The Macmillan Companu.

Greysen, S., Chen, C., & Mullan, F. (2011). A history of medical student debt: Observations and implications for the future of medical education. *Academic Medicine, 86*(7), 840–845.

Hammoud, M., Nuthalapaty, F., Goepfert, A., Casey, P., Emmons, S., Espey, E., . . . Association of Professors of Gynecology and Obstet. (2008). To the point: Medical education review of the role of simulators in surgical training. *American Journal of Obstetrics and Gynecology, 199*(4), 338–343.

Hamstra, J., Brydges, R., Hatala, R., Zendejas, B., & Cook, D. (2014). Reconsidering fidelity in simulation-based training. *Academic Medicine, 89*(3), 387–392.

Harasym, P., Woloschuk, W., Mandin, H., & Brundin-Mather, R. (1996). Reliability and validity of interviewers' judgments of medical school candidates. *Academic Medcine, 71*(1), 540–542.

Hoff, T. (2010). *Practice under Presssure: Primary care physicians and their medicine in the twenty-first century.* New Brunswick, NJ: Rutgers University Press.

Holmboe, E., Sherbino, J., Long, D., Swing, S., & Frank, J. (2010). The role of assessment in competency-based medical education. *Medical Teacher, 32*(8), 676–682.

Institute of Medicine (IOM). (1972). *Educating for the health team.* Washington, DC: National Academy of Sciences.

IOM. (1999). *To err is human: Building a safer system.* Washington, DC: National Academy of Sciences.

IOM. (2001). *Crossing the quality chasm: A new health system for the 21st century.* Washington, DC: National Academies Press.

IOM. (2003). *Health professions education: A bridge to quality.* Washington, DC: National Academies Press.

IOM. (2009). *Redesigning continuing education in the health professions.* Washington, DC: National Academies Press.

IOM. (2011). *The future of nursing: Leading change, advancing health.* Washington, DC: National Academies Press.

IOM. (2015). *Measuring the Impact of interprofessional education (IPE) on collaborative practice and patient outcomes.* Washington: National Academies Press.

Interprofessional Education Collaborative Expert Panel. (2011). *Core competencies for interprofessional collaborative practice: Report of an expert panel.* Washington, DC: Interprofessional Education Collaborative.

Jeffe, D., Whelan, A., & Androle, D. (2010). Primary care specialty choices of United States medical graduates, 1997-2006. *Academic Medicine, 85*(6), 947–958.

Joint Commission, The. (April 15, 2014). *Sentinel event data—Root causes by event type.* Retrieved from www.jointcommission.org: http://www.jointcommission.org/sentinel_event_statistics/

Kastor, J. (2011). Accountable care organizations at academic medical centers. *New England Journal of Medicine, 364*, e11.

Khanova, J., Roth, M., Rodgers, J., & McLaughlin, J. (2015). Student experiences across multiple flipped courses in a single curriculum. *Medical Education, 49*(10), 1038–1048.

Khouli, H., Jahnes, K., Shapiro, J., Rose, K., Matthew, J., Gohil, A., . . . Fried, E. (2011). Performance of medical residents in sterile techniques during central vein catheterization: randomized trial of efficacy of simulation-based training. *Chest, 139*(1), 80–87.

King, H., Battles, J., Baker, D., Alonso, A., Salas, E., Webster, J., . . . Salisbury, M. (2008). *TeamSTEPPS: Team Strategies and Tools to Enhance Performance and Patient Safety.* Rockville, MD: Agency for Healthcare Research and Quality.

Lawlis, T., Anson, J., & Greenfield, D. (2014). Barriers and enablers that influence sustainable interprofessional education: a literature review. *Journal of Interprofessional Care, 28*(4), 305–310.

McGaghie, W., Issenberg, S., Barsuk, J., & Wayne, D. (2014). A critical review of simulation-based mastery learning with translational outcomes. *Medical Education, 48*(4), 375–385.

Miller, J., Andersson, G., Cohen, M., Cohen, S., Gibson, S., Hindery, M., . . . Browdy, D. (2012). Follow the money: The implications of medical schools' funds flow models. *Academic Medicine, 87*(12), 1746–1751.

Morgeson, F., DeRue, D., & Karam, E. (2010). Leadership in teams: A functional approach to understanding leadership structures and processes. *Journal of Management, 36*(1), 5–39.

Neily, J., Mills, P., Eldridge, N., Carney, B., Pfeffer, D., Turner, J., . . . Bagian, J. (2011). Incorrect surgical procedures within and outside of the operating room: A follow-up report. *Archives of Surgery, 146*(11), 1235–1239.

Neily, J., Mills, P., Young-Xu, Y., Carney, B., West, P., Berger, D., . . . Bagian, J. (2010). Association between implementation of a medical team training program and surgical mortality. *Journal of the American Medical Association, 304*(15), 1693–1700.

Norman, G., Dore, K., & Grierson, L. (2012). The minimal relationship between simulation fidelity and transfer of learning. *Medical Education, 46*(7), 636–647.

Norris, T., Schaad, D., DeWitt, D., Ogur, B., Hunt, D., & Members of the Consortium of Longitudinal Integration. (2009). Longitudinal integrated clerkships for medical students: An innovation adopted by medical schools in Australia, Canada, South Africa, and the United States. *Academic Medicine, 84*(7), 902–907.

Owens, J., & Schmitt, M. (2013). Integrating interprofessional education into continuing education: A planning process for continuing interprofessional education programs. *Journal of Continuing Education in the Health Professions, 33*(2), 109–117.

Reeves, S. (2012). The rise and rise of interprofessional competence. *Journal of Interprofessional Care, 26*(4), 253–255.

Reeves, S., Lewin, S., Espin, S., & Zwarenstein, M. (2010). *Interprofessional teamwork for health and social care.* Oxford, UK: Wiley-Blackwell.

Reeves, S., Perrier, L., Goldman, J., Freeth, D., & Zwarenstein, M. (2013). Interprofessional education: Effects on professional practice and healthcare outcomes (update). *Cochrane Database of Systematic Reviews, 3,* CD002213.

Reeves, S., Zwarenstein, M., Goldman, J., Barr, H., Freeth, D., Hammick, M., & Koppel, I. (2008). Interprofessional education: effects on professional practice and health care outcomes. *The Cochrane Collaboration and Database of Systemic Reviews,* CD002213.

Salas, E., DiazGranados, D., Klein, C., Burke, C., Stagl, K., Goodwin, G., & Halpin, S. (2008). Does team training improve team performance? A meta-analysis. *Human Factors: The Journal of the Human Factors and Ergonomics, 50*(6), 903–933.

Salas, E., Gregory, M., & King, H. (2011). Team training can enhance patient safety—the data, the challenge ahead. *Joint Commission Journal of Quality and Patient Safety, 37*(8), 339–340.

Schumacher, D., Englander, R., & Carraccio, C. (2013). Developing the master learner: Applying learning theory to the learner, the teacher, and the learning environment. *Academic Medicine, 88*(11), 1635–1645.

Sitkin, S., & Sutcliffe, K. (1991). Dispensing legitimacy: Professional, organizational, and legal influences on pharmacist behavior. *Research in the Sociology of Organizations, 8,* 269–295.

Starr, P. (1982). *The social transformation of American medicine.* New York, NY: Basic Books.

Teherani, A., Irby, D., & Loeser, H. (2013). Outcomes of different clerkship models: Longitudinal integrated, hybrid, and block. *Academic Medicine, 88*(1), 35–43.

Walsh, K. (2015). The costs of clinical education. *Medical Teacher, 37*(7), 605–607.

Walters, L., Greenhill, J., Richards, J., Ward, H., Campbell, N., Ash, J., & Schuwirth, L. (2012). Outcomes of longitudinal integrated clinical placements for students, clinicians and society. *Medical Education, 46*(11), 1028–1041.

White, K., Williams, T., & Greenberg, B. (1961). The ecology of medical care. *New England Journal of Medicine, 265,* 885–892.

Wolf, S., Lockspeiser, T., Gong, J., & Guiton, G. (2014). Students' perspectives on the fourth year of medical school: A mixed-methods analysis. *Academic Medicine, 89,* 602–607.

Woloschuk, W., Myhre, D., Jackson, W., McLaughlin, K., & Wright, B. (2014). Comparing the performance in family medicine residencies of graduates from longitudinal integrated clerkships and rotation-based clerkships. *Academic Medicine, 89*(2), 296–300.

World Health Organization. (2010). *Framework for action on interprofessional education and collaborative practice.* Geneva: World Health Organization.

Zanedjas, B., Wang, A., Brydges, R., Hamstra, S., & Cook, D. (2013). Cost: The missing outcome in simulation-based medical education research: A systematic review. *Surgery, 153*(2), 160–176.

Zorek, J., & Raehl, C. (2013). Interprofessional education accreditation standards in the USA: A comparative analysis. *Journal of Interprofessional Care, 27*(2), 123–130.

COMMENTARY TO ACCOMPANY CHAPTER 6

George Thibault

THE CHAPTER BY Alan Dow and Scott Reeves highlights a number of important trends for health professional education in the 21st century with the goal of better preparing the future health professions workforce for an evolving healthcare system. These trends include interprofessional education (IPE), a competency rather than a time-based approach to education, new models for clinical education such as the longitudinal integrated clerkship, and increasing use of educational technology.

The recrudescence of the interest in IPE is an acknowledgment of the fact that healthcare professionals will work in teams (variously defined and variously formed) throughout their careers. Therefore, an understanding of other health professions and the acquisition of team-based skills should be part of the educational goals for all health professionals. It is well known that there are many logistical and cultural barriers to accomplishing IPE, but there are now an increasing number of examples of successful IPE programs involving students of nursing, medicine, and other health professions (Josiah Macy Jr. Foundation, 2012). The authors are correct in pointing out that much more work needs to be done to assess these programs in order to learn the appropriate "dose" of IPE—in what settings, with what interprofessional partners, and at what time in the educational continuum. The ultimate goal, of course, is to show that educational interventions such as IPE can lead to better patient outcomes, and to this end the National Center for Interprofessional

Practice and Education has been created as a unique public/private partnership (National Center for Interprofessional Practice and Education, n.d.).

Another trend is a competency-based approach to education in the health professions, which could shorten the time (and therefore the cost) of education. Even more important, a competency-based educational process would more securely satisfy our professional obligation to assure the public of the readiness of graduates to move along their professional trajectories. Pursuing this goal for physician training, there are programs now exploring shorter, competency-based paths to the degree of Doctor of Medicine (Josiah Macy Jr. Foundation, n.d.a) and others, combining undergraduate and graduate education in certain disciplines (Josiah Macy Jr. Foundation, n.d.b). As the authors point out, research is needed to establish rigorous and testable competencies across the professions.

Because more care is moving out of the hospital into other settings and because most health professionals will be involved primarily in the management of chronic disease over time, there is a need for new models of clinical education that reflect this changing site of care and changing burdens of disease. The longitudinal integrated clerkship for medical students is one such model, which is based on the principle of continuity—continuity of patients, continuity of teachers, continuity of site, and continuity of curriculum (Hirsh, Ogur, Thibault, & Cox, 2007). Other new models will be required to prepare a range of health professionals for the care of different patient populations in different settings.

A fourth trend is the use of new and developing educational technologies to facilitate changes in education in the health professions and increase the efficiency and accessibility of the educational process. For example, both simulation and online learning can help overcome some of the logistical barriers to IPE. The "flipped classroom" can increase the efficiency of information transfer and allow precious faculty and student time together to be spent in achieving other educational goals such as critical thinking, teamwork, communication, and professionalism. Appropriately used, educational and information technologies also can help accomplish other educational goals such as a greater individualization of the educational experience, accurate competency assessments, and a tighter link between the education of health professionals and patient and population clinical data (Josiah Macy Jr. Foundation, 2015).

In addition to these trends, the authors comment on some very important themes that are cross-cutting. The first of these is the need to more closely link changes in education for the health professions with changes in healthcare delivery. This was echoed in the recommendations of a recent Macy conference, which stated the principle that "educational reform must incorporate practice redesign and delivery system change must include a central education mission if we are to achieve enduring transformation" (Josiah Macy Jr. Foundation, 2013).

A second theme is the need to focus more on the educational continuum of all health professions from prelicensure education to continuing professional development during a career in practice. This framework enables one to think of competencies that are appropriate at each stage and to see the educational process (for each profession and across the professions) as a lifelong process rather than a series of discrete endpoints. Finally, implicit in all this is the need for more educational research to establish the relationship between educational interventions and better patient outcomes and better functioning of the healthcare system.

The overall thrust of this excellent chapter is that we need better alignment of education for health professionals with the changing needs of a 21st-century patient population and healthcare system. That will require innovation, leadership, and research. It also will require that we invest in the next generation of health professional educators who will lead this innovation (Josiah Macy Jr. Foundation, n.d.c).

References

Hirsh, D. A., Ogur, B., Thibault, G. E., & Cox, M. (2007). New models of clinical clerkships: "Continuity" as an organizing principle for clinical education reform. *New England Journal of Medicine 356*(8), 858–866.

Josiah Macy Jr. Foundation. (2015). Proceedings on a conference on enhancing health professions education through technology: Building a continuously learning health system, April 9–12. Available from: http://macyfoundation.org/publications/publication/ enhancing-health-professions-education-through-technology

Josiah Macy Jr. Foundation. (2012). Proceedings on a conference on interprofessional education, April 1–3. Available from: http://macyfoundation.org/docs/macy_pubs/JMF_IPE_book_ web.pdf

Josiah Macy Jr. Foundation. (2013). Proceedings on a conference on transforming patient care: aligning interprofessional education with clinical practice redesign, January 17–20. Available from: http://macyfoundation.org/docs/macy_pubs/JMF_ TransformingPatientCare_Jan2013Conference_fin_Web.pdf

Josiah Macy Jr. Foundation. n.d.a. Grant to New York University. (February 2015–January 2019). Consortium of medical schools with accelerated pathways programs. http://macyfoundation. org/grantees/profile/consortium-of-medical-schools-with-accelerated-pathway-programs

Josiah Macy Jr. Foundation. n.d.b. Grant to the Association of American Medical Colleges. (July 2013–June 2016). Education in pediatrics across the continuum—a competency-based medical education pilot. http://macyfoundation.org/grantees/profile/ consortium-of-medical-schools-with-accelerated-pathway-programs

Josiah Macy Jr. Foundation. n.d.c. Macy Faculty Scholars: About the program. (New York, NY). Available from: http://macyfoundation.org/docs/macy_pubs/JMF_FacultyScholars_Brochure_2016_Web.pdf

National Center for Interprofessional Practice and Education. n.d. Home page. (Minneapolis, MN). https://nexusipe.org/

7

IMPLICATIONS OF PROFESSIONAL CHANGE FOR HEALTH

POLICY, PRACTICE, AND MANAGEMENT

*Timothy J. Hoff, Kathleen M. Sutcliffe, and Gary J. Young**

Introduction

"Change never starts, because it never stops" (Weick & Quinn, 1999). This maxim certainly captures the turmoil faced by health professions over the past several decades. But as disruptive as the past has been, the sum of this book's chapters suggests that it has only been a prelude to current and future transformations. Things indeed are in flux. In this final chapter, we summarize the "things" that collectively stand out.

The convergence of perspectives and ideas across chapters that were produced independently of one another is striking. Chapter authors emphasize a common set of conceptual similarities, issues, and recurring themes. The chapters in this volume in many ways interrelate and reinforce one another, so much so that we have a real sense of emerging themes and theoretical issues. This may simply be coincidence. Alternatively, it may reflect a growing synthesis of perception and understanding, bringing into focus what has been until now a set of blurred images. We find this convergence somewhat surprising given the complexity and dynamism of the healthcare professions.

---

* All authors contributed equally to the chapter and are listed alphabetically.

In this final chapter, we discuss these key emergent themes, their associated theoretical and conceptual considerations, key implications for practice and patient care, and select gaps and questions the book does not address that remain important. As noted in Chapter 1, in this book we are not concerned with doing an exhaustive treatment of all the major changes occurring in the US healthcare professional workforce. Our intention has been to sample in a critical way some key areas of transformation, innovation, and change. In this chapter, we take a similar stance, focusing on emerging themes and their associated implications for both health professions and the US health system.

Theme: The Increased Shifting and Blurring of Professional Boundaries

A key theme emerging from across the chapters is the increased shifting and blurring of professional boundaries within the US healthcare system. As this book has described, important changes are pushing specific professional work domains in new and different directions. There are external developments involving the increased aging and morbidity of our population, particularly in the area of chronic disease (Centers for Disease Control and Prevention [CDC], 2014). This has driven up the demand for services, for example, producing more than a billion outpatient visits (CDC, 2016). An older, sicker population has strained the system's ability to provide timely, accessible care. In addition, the almost 17 million newly insured individuals produced by the Affordable Care Act has resulted in further problems on the demand side. These realities have illuminated the lack of physicians in key areas of medicine such as primary care, spurring the need for innovation regarding who delivers services and how those services are delivered.

These innovations, ranging from the increased standardization of care through the use of guidelines and electronic health record technology, to the use of collaborative teams to deliver care, to global forms of payment that reward lower-cost care delivery offer nurses, physician assistants, and other professionals opportunities to expand their interactions with patients and gain increased exposure to independent clinical work. This furthers the legitimacy of nonphysician professionals with the public and physicians, enabling them to advance causes such as more complex training, higher salaries, and enhanced freedoms to practice independently. Physicians, moving through profound changes of their own, as detailed by Hoff and Pohl in Chapter 2, may be more amenable than ever before to sharing some of their power and authority over care delivery due in part to the increased complexity of managing care, their limited capacities for taking on any additional work, and shifts in their own values and expectations. For example, many younger physicians view their profession as a good "8 to 5" job within which they are willing to trade a greater emphasis on lifestyle concerns in return for letting their employing organizations make more of the care structuring decisions, decisions that include the greater use of non-physician professionals and sharing of authority. As Spetz, Cawley, and Schommer point out in Chapter 3, the latter groups wish to upskill and do more, and so they increasingly find themselves within political and clinical environments that support those goals.

Thus, as healthcare work changes, and as larger healthcare systems move into positions of prominence in making key decisions about how various workflows of importance should be organized, there is a commensurate impact on professional work domains and increased acknowledgment that professional work boundaries should be more fluid, interconnected, and permeable. The consumer engagement movement in healthcare, described by Hoff, Sutcliffe, and Young in Chapter 1, also facilitates this general trend. An important component of this movement seeks to emphasize more than simply the physician-patient interaction specifically when considering the patient's total experience in a healthcare transaction. It also seeks to root out waste in all its forms from various healthcare workflows. In part, this means doing more with lower-cost professional labor. The impact that consumer engagement thinking is having on many in the industry involves a greater consideration of the different ways healthcare services might be provided to patients and of how to maximize a satisfying experience for the healthcare customer. This line of thinking suggests that no one professional has the exclusive corner on creating this type of experience and that healthcare teams of different professionals with meaningful responsibilities likely can deliver enhanced value better.

As the chapters in this book note, health professionals of all types are developing shared interests, even if some do not yet realize it fully, as they find themselves doing their work in larger organizations that have the scale and negotiating power to compete effectively for care delivery dollars, insurance premiums, and other financial rewards. As the chapters also note, these shared interests are slowly but surely affecting areas such as professional training (e.g., interprofessional training), care delivery (e.g., team care), organizational governance (e.g., conjoint and hybrid leadership structures), and talent management (e.g., job and benefit design). Next, we make several additional observations that emerge from the boundary shifting theme.

THE END OF PHYSICIAN DOMINANCE?

Does the shifting and blurring of professional boundaries in healthcare signal the end of "physician dominance" (Freidson, 1970)? Probably not, but it certainly signals an increased era of "physician compromise." No longer does the medical profession have the sort of influence and control it once did over key aspects of the system involving payment, quality, or clinical decision-making. That said, the profession continues to retain a great deal of authority over how healthcare is organized and delivered, as Chapters 2, 4, and 5 all point out. Increasingly, this reality will also change. For example, if team-based care evolves as a viable means to organize many aspects of healthcare service delivery, physicians will need (and may want) to partner more as coequals with other team members such as nurses, physician assistants, social workers, and physical therapists. Chapters 2 and 3 talk about this reality, as does Chapter 6 in terms of how it will affect professional training. As physicians perhaps have less direct face time with their patients, and those patients have more engagement with other health professionals, the views and experiential knowledge possessed by the latter groups will become important to heed and act on. These front-line providers will become valuable sources for understanding how patient care should be delivered. At a macro level, physician influence will be tempered in areas such as primary care by healthcare corporations pushing nonphysician-based models of care delivery.

Interesting research questions here could focus on better understanding which types of compromises physicians are likely to embrace and how those compromises might shape key system outcomes such as the cost of care, the nature of professional training, features of healthcare quality, and the organization of clinical workflows. Conceptually, it will behoove the field to develop ideas that focus on interprofessional symbiosis and mutual interdependence that more accurately map onto what is happening within everyday healthcare practice. Studying and theorizing about professional work and interactions in new ways also becomes imperative, as traditional perspectives and research built around separateness of professional work domains and physician power become less informative. Practically, a key management imperative becomes how to bring different health professionals together in ways that minimize conflict and maximize their ability to work as collectives in efficient ways—sharing some of the same work, making decisions jointly, and working within structures where power is more dispersed among the stakeholders.

THE RISE OF A VIGOROUS INTERPROFESSIONAL SOLIDARITY?

The increased presence of shared interests among health professionals raises a host of interesting topics for further investigation that have both theoretical and practical significance. One topic involves the potential for joint collective action on the part of physicians, nurses, and others. This is a topic not addressed in any of this book's chapters. Yet it is absolutely suggested by the types of professional dynamics Chapter 2 discusses in relation to physicians, Chapter 3 in relation to nurses and pharmacists, and Chapter 6 in relation to the benefits of greater interprofessional training and socialization.

Several years ago during the managed care era, the issue of whether or not US physicians might embrace unionization (Hoff, 2005) gained traction. Meanwhile, nurses and other health professionals have been organizing collectively for years. The notion of physicians engaging in collective action such as strikes and contract bargaining alongside other professionals is not as far-fetched as it used to be, and physicians in other health systems, including the United Kingdom's National Health Service, are no strangers to the use of collective action (Triggle, 2016). Interesting investigative foci here include identifying the types of issues (e.g., pay, working conditions) for which physicians might unite with other health professionals to bargain collectively and the types of outcomes obtained through the kinds of bargaining that might involve multiple groups of professionals simultaneously.

Practically, healthcare organizations have a strategic interest in understanding the shared interests that may exist across professional groups. For instance, given issues related to lower levels of job satisfaction and higher burnout across all health professionals, the ability to create work environments that possess qualities equally important to all these workers enhances the prospects for more effective professional recruitment and retention and does so efficiently. It is increasingly important to identify and address the similarities that exist among different health professional groups in terms of job design, work outcomes such as job satisfaction, career development, and continuing education. In this way, healthcare organizations can develop holistic rather than piecemeal approaches to talent management.

Finally, the increased interprofessional homogeneity of interests forces professional associations to reflect on how they seek to advance their particular constituency's causes. Such associations may become more collaborative in the future, innovating their lobbying and advocacy approaches in ways that enhance their collective leverage vis-à-vis healthcare employers. This heightens the possibilities for driving preferred changes both in the system at large and their members' everyday workplaces.

THE CONTINUED EVOLUTION OF HEALTHCARE WORK?

We are in a period where the shifting and blurring of professional work boundaries will continue. This means that the very nature of work in the health professions will keep changing. For example, as alluded to in Chapter 3, some nursing work may become more like some physician work, as many nurses become more involved in direct patient care, particularly in primary care. Some physician work may become less "hands on" and more distal from the individual patient, as physicians' specific skills are used increasingly in a consulting or population health management capacity. Different individuals within the same profession, as Chapter 2 describes with respect to physicians, will gravitate toward work that best fits their personalities, interests, and experience. More generally, the image of the single expert interacting with the single patient could give way to the team of various professionals, each of whom assumes a smaller, more compartmentalized piece of the patient interaction guided by larger quality and efficiency goals. In short, what it means to be a "physician," "nurse," or "pharmacist" will keep changing, and roles will become more diverse. In part, this will also occur because features of the work health care professionals are asked to do keep changing and the workflows within which they find themselves are continually overhauled.

Conceptually, this evolution raises the question of whether and how we should make generalizations about professional work, particularly in healthcare. Traditional theories on professions fixate on ideal or typical categorizations of "profession" and "professional," emphasizing, for example, qualities such as discretion, autonomy, and control over a specific work jurisdiction as universal traits (Freidson, 1970; Abbott, 1988). But in a fluid environment where different groups of health professionals frequently acquire, give up, and negotiate various qualities of their work and identity, what use can such generalizations serve to explain how these groups of workers self-identify, behave, or relate to clients and other colleagues?

Imagine the pathways to laying claim to a specific professional work domain become more grounded in contextual circumstances such as workforce shortages, innovation implementation, consumer engagement, or changes in the structural environment such as payment, as alluded to throughout the prior chapters. Then we will need fresh approaches to theorizing about professionals and their work, rooted in perspectives that emphasize both the evolutionary and contingent natures of what it means to think and act like a specific type of healthcare professional. In addition, predicting which work domains end up the purview of which health professionals in the future will become an exercise for not only understanding the strategic imperatives and system needs that must be met, but also understanding how professions themselves attempt to compete with each other and gain control over particular types of work.

A TRULY MORE PATIENT-CENTRIC HEALTHCARE SYSTEM—AS PROFESSIONALS DEFINE IT?

One might imagine that a shifting and blurring of professional boundaries in healthcare could also affect patient care in significant ways. How could this play out? One school of thought is that the very notion of patient-centered care is shaped primarily through the application of organizational policies and management practices that seek to gain greater input directly from patients about their needs, expectations, and preferences. A second related perspective is that it is the industry's responsibility, through the application of consumer engagement principles, to help patients identify their needs and preferences; in the process, these desires are shaped in ways that lead to better business relationships between individual customers and healthcare organizations.

But a more integrated professional work sphere, and the collective action it intimates, could place healthcare professionals at the forefront of defining what patient centrism means and how to act on it. One area of investigation in this regard could look at how the very manifestation of patient-centric care, for example, might look different than what we are seeing now. Imagine groups of collaborative health professionals who work, train, and govern together (and also share similar patient care and work interests) take the lead as a combined force in pushing for their own unique vision of such a concept. Instead of standardized metrics presumed to be patient-friendly in providing transparency and comparability being at the center of healthcare quality, would health professionals instead advocate for greater emphasis on the relational aspects of care in which interpersonal qualities such as trust between patient and provider take center stage? Would a turn toward these relational aspects make more patients more satisfied regarding their care experiences or more likely to become involved in their own health maintenance?

From a practice perspective, one might imagine the impact a professionally guided patient-centric approach would have on the health workplace. Innovations such as electronic medical records, which in their current form are anathema to many professionals, might be deemphasized in the provision of care. Workflow design in clinical care delivery could move from a core emphasis on transactional speed and reducing "waste" to greater relational development between staff and patients that emphasizes interaction quality and time spent together. In short, it is possible to imagine a pushback against the current forces aimed at standardizing care delivery. Of course, the professional perspective on patient centrism could run headlong into the realities of how physicians and healthcare organizations now need to earn revenue to survive and compete. Or, alternatively, it could shift parts of the current system in directions that over the long term produce a delivery system that seems more personally appealing to both the workers and customers alike. In any event, the blurring of professional work and role boundaries offer a renewed opportunity for the healthcare system to engage a meaningful collective voice in the debate about (a) how healthcare should be structured and (b) what patients should receive in the process. This is not a bad thing.

Theme: Increased Alignment Between Health Professionals and Organizations

A second central theme that emerges in the book is the importance of increased alignment between healthcare organizations and health professionals, resulting in better patient care. As noted in several chapters, the lack of symbiosis between the two entities with respect to the delivery of healthcare services has been a long-standing problem. From the chapters, we glean three key interrelated considerations for moving toward greater alignment between the two parties.

One consideration is the need for innovation in the way relationships between healthcare organizations and health professionals are structured. Alexander and Young in Chapter 4, in particular, call for greater flexibility in the types of business and financial arrangements that exist between these parties. They emphasize, as do Noordegraaf and Burns in Chapter 5, the value of more shared governance arrangements overall between health professionals and healthcare organizations for patient care decision-making but also contend that neither salaried employment nor looser forms of affiliation will be the best universal approach for achieving alignment. So while the current trend, as Hoff and Pohl in Chapter 2 point out, is toward the direct employment of physicians by hospitals and healthcare systems, it remains to be seen whether putting physicians directly on the payroll is a highly effective approach by healthcare organizations for achieving alignment. However, what arrangements are good alternatives and when they merit use is not well understood, a point that comes across in several of the chapters. Innovation and experimentation are sorely needed in this regard.

A second consideration involves the ability of healthcare organizations to manage collaborative relationships among different types of health professionals. The insularity of various professional groups has been a defining feature of US healthcare organizations, one which healthcare organizations historically have at least passively accepted if not in some cases actively supported. This reality is now juxtaposed with calls from the health policy community for greater intra- and interprofessional collaboration as an important element for achieving tighter linkages between healthcare organizations and health professionals.

Noordegraaf and Burns express strong reservations about the ability of healthcare organizations to meet this challenge, given what they see as significant differences in cultural identity among health professional groups. This challenge for healthcare organizations is complicated by changing scopes of practice among some health professionals. Several chapters, most notably Chapter 3 by Spetz, Cawley, and Schommer, explain that regulatory and educational reforms for health professionals such as nurse practitioners and pharmacists are expanding their scopes of practice, resulting in overlapping clinical domains among other such professionals and with primary care physicians. Healthcare organizations will need to confront this issue in their efforts to manage interprofessional collaboration, because collaboration could give way to competition. However, we noted earlier that there is increased shifting and blurring of professional work in healthcare, and this trend will continue. This may provide additional opportunities for healthcare organizations to assist various professional groups in their attempts to become more integrated and, in the process, afford them an opportunity to align their interests with those of these groups.

A third consideration involves training of health professionals. Several chapters indicate that greater alignment requires that health professionals possess knowledge and skills that fall outside the scope of traditional forms of professional education. Such knowledge and skills include participating on interdisciplinary clinical teams, providing patient care to meet performance metrics for both quality and efficiency, and developing services for promoting population health. In Chapter 6, Dow and Reeves outline some of the educational reforms that academic institutions are undertaking to better prepare health professionals to meet the challenges of today's workforce requirements.

Still, fully preparing health professionals for the varied skills and competencies they must use in a reformed health system seems a tall order for academic institutions, one that may realistically exceed what can be accomplished within the time frames of conventional academic training for professionals such as physicians and nurses. As such, it may be that future health professionals will enter the workforce with substantial gaps in needed knowledge and skills.

These considerations raise a number of interesting research questions. In particular, under what circumstances should healthcare organizations employ health professionals versus contract with them to efficiently achieve alignment about patient care goals? This question provides for fascinating study, particularly as new types of organizations such as accountable care organizations and retail clinics step forward with their own ideas for achieving alignment. Some theoretical perspectives (e.g., Tadelis, 2002) consider this type of decision to be largely a matter of whether the contract-related costs (e.g., performance monitoring and enforcement) that healthcare organizations would face in securing the services of certain types of health professionals are foreseeable and controllable. If not, employment is likely to be the preferred approach. But such perspectives may be too narrowly focused for addressing this question given the cultural barriers that have long prevented healthcare organizations and health professionals from collaborating more effectively together to improve patient care, barriers which have been outlined in previous chapters of this book. Another question for future research is what are the most effective ways for an organization to integrate different groups of health professionals, whether employed or under contract, into its strategic and clinical decision-making processes to achieve interprofessional collaboration?

Although more research is needed to help healthcare organizations sort out the answers to these questions, existing evidence already suggests that these organizations should not approach issues of alignment entirely or even largely in terms of business and financial considerations, which in the past has typically been the case. For organizations to secure the loyalty of their workforce members, professionals included, they should treat them beneficially in ways that are often unrelated to financial compensation such as in matters of work autonomy, effective communication, or professional development. A recent study suggests that when healthcare organizations provide such beneficial treatment to their health professionals, the professionals more closely identify with their affiliated healthcare organization and are also more likely to comply with requested management initiatives (e.g., Hekman, Bigley, Steensma, & Hereford, 2009).

PRACTICAL CONSIDERATIONS FOR ACHIEVING PROFESSIONAL–ORGANIZATIONAL ALIGNMENT

Although many uncertainties exist as to how healthcare organizations and health professionals will work through the alignment issues noted above, the book directly or indirectly points to a number of practice-related action items that are important to consider.

First, whatever ways healthcare organizations and health professions choose to affiliate with one another, healthcare organizations should remain sensitive to the full range of similarities and differences in work-related preferences and attitudes among their health professional groups. A one-size arrangement may not fit all, but there will be arrangements that can satisfy more than single professional groups simultaneously. This comes across clearly in Chapter 2 by Hoff and Pohl, who speak specifically to evolving relations between physicians and healthcare organizations. They observe the growing stratification of the medical profession along the lines of age, gender, and specialization and its implications for increasing diversity among physicians with respect to topics such as career development, job and workplace design, and work–life balance.

Second, healthcare organizations should be prepared to assume a greater role in helping to define scopes of practice for health professionals, which, as explained above and throughout the book, will remain fluid for some time. Although Spetz, Cawley, and Schommer in Chapter 3 anticipate that relevant regulatory agencies will work together to update professional practice regulations to address overlapping scopes of practice among health professionals, it seems just as likely that these agencies will move slowly or not at all in addressing this issue. If so, healthcare organizations may have more latitude to define their own scopes of practice for health professionals that focus on their strategic objectives rather than meeting licensure and accreditation requirements. Healthcare organizations should consider being proactive to leverage this opportunity to build cooperation among their health professionals around newly defined clinical roles as part of the clinical architecture that supports interprofessional collaboration. In essence, we could see a move toward the privatization of professional practice regulation. Noordegraaf and Burns, in Chapter 5, also offer some valuable proposals for shared clinical governance arrangements that healthcare organizations can adopt to define their own scopes of practice.

Third, there is an expanded role for healthcare organizations in educating health professionals. As noted, it seems likely that traditional professional educational systems and the academic institutions in which they are housed will be unable to fully prepare health professionals for the full scope of realities, challenges, and work requirements that lie ahead of them in today's work environments. In Chapter 6, Dow and Reeves invoke such concern by noting important gaps in current training curricula such as getting young health professionals ready to participate in formalized team structures for patient care delivery. Healthcare organizations may fill some of this void.

Hoff and Pohl in Chapter 2 allude to this in considering opportunities for healthcare organizations to address the changing talent management needs of the future physician workforce. The previously noted possibility that healthcare organizations will have more say in specifying scopes of practice for health professionals makes this all the more compelling; one implication is that clinical positions for health professionals will be less standardized, and thus more on the job training will be needed. Although healthcare organizations have in the past offered some educational training for health professionals, including the development of mentorship programs, the need for organizations to expand their own training for professionals will likely increase dramatically. This increase may be so great that entry-level and continuing education for health professionals may someday become a source of competitive advantage for healthcare organizations in recruitment and retention activities. The recent announcement by Kaiser Permanente, a national provider of managed healthcare, that it will be opening its own medical school seems entirely consistent with this perspective (Rovner, 2015).

Theme: Increasing Diversity and Differentiation

Themes of diversity, differentiation, and more generally, variation, are prominent throughout the book, and we have touched on some of them in earlier sections. Still, the sway of diversity is so important and so overarching that we take the liberty to single it out here. The term *diversity* can provoke negative reactions. We use it here to mean simply "variety" or a "point or respect in which things differ" (Houghton Mifflin Company, 1993, p. 369). For example, Chapter 1 describes a variety of exogenous and endogenous forces fueling health profession transformation. Chapters 2 and 3 clearly focus on diversity, differentiation, and stratification within professions (e.g., gender, expertise, work roles, practice settings). Chapters 4 and 5 describe variety in the more macro organizational arrangements at play in healthcare systems and organizations, as well as the diverse set of microsystem practices aimed at leading and managing health professionals. Finally, Chapter 6 explores increasing diversity in required professional skills and competencies and the educational approaches used to assure them.

Just as America's population is becoming increasingly diverse, so too is the healthcare workforce, especially medicine, pharmacy, and physician assistants. A common way to distinguish diversity is with respect to (a) observable or readily detectable attributes such as gender and age and (b) less visible or underlying attributes such as values, personality characteristics, expertise, and technical abilities. Diversity in health professions is increasing along both dimensions. As Hoff and Pohl point out in Chapter 2, the percentage of women in medicine has increased significantly—30% of the US physician workforce now is female, and almost 50% of the applicants to medical school are female.

In addition to an historical predominance of female nurse practitioners, Spetz, Cawley and Schommer point out in Chapter 3 that women now compose 66% of working physician assistants and more than 50% of licensed pharmacists. In some professions such as medicine and physician assistants, gender diversity is accompanied by increased age diversity and an increase rise in younger providers. Younger providers have different world views, value systems, and job expectations than their older counterparts. These differences shape their perspectives on current transformations in the healthcare industry as well as their career expectations and motivations.

For example, Hoff and Pohl suggest that younger physicians increasingly value a work–life balance. They are much more likely to trade autonomy for a more stable, personally appealing lifestyle, meaning that they are more comfortable with ceding particular aspects of the work and decision-making to other professional groups (e.g., nurse practitioners, physician assistants, pharmacists), patients, and to their employing organizations (e.g., working as salaried employees for larger organizations that can shoulder nonclinical responsibilities). Moreover, they may be faster and more facile at adopting new technologies and new ways of working (e.g., care pathways, clinical teams) that can contribute to different types of patient interactions and outcomes.

In addition to increasing diversity in terms of individual demographics and attributes, intraprofessional diversity is increasing related to clinical specialization and increased variation in career opportunities and work roles. These changes are a result of upskilling and other forces such as changes in the more general structure of healthcare systems, changes in societal demands of healthcare (i.e., value, quality, safety), and advances in science and technology. Specialization in medicine is rampant. As Chapter 2 notes, there are now more than 120 medical specialties. Also, as Chapter 3 notes, it is occurring to a lesser extent in nursing and pharmacy. Medicine and pharmacy especially are also experiencing increased variation in career opportunities, work roles, and work practice settings. Certainly, specialization and opportunities for variety in career and work roles may have both task-related and efficiency benefits as professionals become more proficient in performing specialized work and have greater agency over their work. These transformations also can increase overall job satisfaction by improving job fit in the sense of better matching people's competencies and interests to their work.

But intraprofessional diversity in the form of increased work specialization may also widen within-profession fault lines for two reasons. Some specialties may compete and work at cross purposes, and in some (as highlighted in Chapter 2) specialties, work roles, and work settings are privileged and deemed more valuable or of higher status than others. Even the field of nursing is experiencing this phenomenon, as it seeks to ascribe higher prestige to nurse practitioners versus registered nurses. Excessive specialization can also adversely and directly affect patient care outcomes if it results in care duplication on the one hand, or fragmentation, gaps in care coordination, and higher costs on the other.

In fact, several important diversity-related theoretical perspectives are relevant for thinking through the potential consequences of this increasing variety among health professionals. What is clear from this work is that researchers must go beyond assessing a single dimension of diversity and pay more attention to the specific contours of diversity and its differential effects within particular units, teams, or groups. We noted that gender diversity (and to some extent age diversity) is increasing within the health professions. To understand diversity's effects, particularly the effects of readily detected attributes (e.g., visible ones such as gender and relative age), it is useful to turn to ideas about social identity and social categorization (see Williams & O'Reilly, 1998).

Studies show that demographic attributes such as gender and age often represent peoples' values, beliefs, and attitudes and are likely to shape their interpersonal relationships. The basic idea is that when people perceive similarities between themselves and others, they are more likely and more strongly to identify with them and to develop more positive feelings about them. And the opposite holds true as well.

When people perceive dissimilarities between themselves and others, they are less likely to identify with them and more likely to experience negative affective reactions to them. The upshot is that groups composed of people who are different from each other are more likely to experience relational conflict or difficulties with social integration, communication, and other social processes such as cooperation. These untoward dynamics indirectly influence outcomes (i.e., teamwork, care coordination, even patient outcomes) through their effects on social relations and group processes.

In contrast, we know that diversity in less visible "task-oriented attributes" such as education, tenure, work-role experience, or functional background are often associated with knowledge, skills and abilities and thought to have a more direct (and more positive) bearing on performance (Jackson, Joshi, & Erhardt, 2003). That is, a group composed of various experts is more likely to develop better (and more innovative) solutions to complex problems, which can lead to better outcomes. Although the past several decades have seen intensive efforts to understand how workplace diversity influences team and organizational functioning, there are few conclusive findings. This makes it even more difficult to predict how things might play out in highly distributed, loosely coupled healthcare contexts. A push for greater use of team models of care, however, demands attention to better understanding the potential effects of these sources of diversity in healthcare. In this way, we may see how to create more positive intra- and intergroup relations.

Several chapters highlight increases in intraprofessional stratification and differentiation. We noted earlier some potential benefits of these transformations. However, there also may be some negative effects. It can weaken professional solidarity. This may contribute to changes in the distribution of power and legitimacy of particular roles within professions or to disproportionate changes in the power and influence of particular specialties (especially in medicine). As we noted in an earlier section, these changes may fuel efforts to collectively organize or unionize. Of course, changes in stratification are being accompanied by overall growth of women in the health professions more generally. This shift in what historically have been male-dominated environments (e.g., physician assistants, pharmacists) may serve to confound our understanding of the underlying dynamics at play and their potential ramifications.

Naturally, an important question to ask is: what happens overall to an industry with an increasingly female workforce? Chapter 2 by Hoff and Pohl in particular discusses some of the potential implications of a significantly female US medical profession. Nursing already is such a profession, with an overwhelming proportion of women. Understanding the sticky and persistent issues of gender inequality may be one way to better understand the potential implications for professions with heavy doses of female membership. But that inequality in many ways arises from more widely held sociocultural beliefs about what is appropriate behavior in a society. Social role theory explains how broader sociocultural beliefs among individuals about the appropriate roles and abilities of men and women can have widespread effects in the workplace (Joshi, 2014). Gender acts as a cue to identify a person's skills and abilities. When women hold roles that are atypical to cultural norms, they are deemed less capable and their contributions are discounted or undervalued. This may explain why the educational gains made by women in science and engineering have not led to the same gains in the science and engineering workplaces (Joshi, 2014). The precise way these dynamics are playing out among health professions is unclear and needs more study. As Hoff and Pohl note in reference to medicine, there exist questions of assimilation versus transformation with respect to greater gender diversity in the medical workplace that bear watching.

The above discussion highlights some of the positive as well as negative consequences of diversity. But an important practical question for healthcare organizations is: how might we manage such diversity? The typical answer is for organizations to undertake a variety of initiatives—the most common being individual inclusion or sensitivity training. Diversity training generally is targeted at individual attitudes (e.g., stereotypes and biases) and behaviors (e.g., relational competencies), and it has been shown to be a somewhat effective method for improving sensitivity and inclusion (Bezrukova & Jehn, 2001). However, a focus on individuals ignores the important social dynamics that develop within organizations, work units, or work teams. Thus, effective diversity management may require more extensive changes in organizational policies, practices, and cultures (Jackson et al., 2003). Culture is acquired through social learning and socialization processes; it is learned over time as groups solve problems. Culture is also a function of the stability of the group as well as the length of time that it has existed. Changing culture in open, distributed healthcare organizations and systems, where providers often assemble in particular contexts and are only loosely coupled, is challenging. At a minimum, organizations can attempt to promote positive intergroup relations by designing interventions that encourage repeated positive interactions among dissimilar groups.

Interestingly, nowhere in this book is mention made of changing cultural diversity, particularly along racial and ethnic lines or the associated implications. Policymakers for decades have argued that to eliminate inequities in the quality and availability of healthcare for underserved populations, the health professional workforce must better reflect the diversity of the patient population. Although the number of providers entering the healthcare workforce who have trained in other countries has increased somewhat over several decades (Zinn & Brannon, 2014), other data (e.g., Institute of Medicine, 2004; O'Neil & the Pew Health Professions

Commission, 1998; Sullivan & the Commission on Diversity in the Healthcare Workforce, 2004) suggest that there has been relatively little progress along these lines. This is a complex problem. One area of future research might be to assess the extent to which universities and academic health centers are working with educational systems to provide elementary and secondary students early exposure to science and health professional populations who are underrepresented in their fields. Anecdotally, there has been some discussion of progress along these lines. However, this progress has yet to show up in dramatically improved rates of racial/ethnic diversity within health professions such as medicine and nursing.

Earlier in this chapter, we highlighted the growing variation in more macro organizational arrangements (e.g., models of care), more micro mechanisms of leading and managing, and increasing variation in educational requirements and methods of teaching and learning. As healthcare organizations and systems struggle to achieve new thresholds of value, lower costs, and higher quality, they demand variety in professional skills, configurations of organizational arrangements, and ways of leading and managing professionals that balance independence with commitment and responsiveness. As we described earlier, there are potential downsides to some aspects of this diversity such as strained relationships between professionals, fragmentation between and among physicians and other professionals, a more confusing delivery system presented to patients, and possible changes in professional power and legitimacy. But there is reason to be hopeful. Consider Ross Ashby's (1958) principle of requisite variety that originated in early systems theory. Ashby suggests that we need variety to control variety; that the internal diversity of any self-regulating system must match the variety and complexity of its environment. Other systems' thinkers such as Haberstroh (1965) describe requisite variety this way "If the environment can disturb a system in a wide variety of ways, then effective control requires a regulator that can sense these disturbances and intervene with a commensurately large repertory of responses" (p. 1176). More recently, Jacqueline Zinn and Diane Brannon (2014) claimed that attention to requisite variety is critical to progress in today's healthcare environments. That is, interventions must be as complex as the challenges they address. Requisite variety reminds us that it may be fruitful to embrace increasing diversity and variation because they are critical to necessary adaptive changes.

Unaddressed Issues and Concluding Thoughts

Although the chapters in this book cover much ground in educating readers about how health professionals, their work, and their work contexts are changing, much has not been discussed. Three issues worthy of note in this regard are: how continued technological innovation in healthcare may affect the future of professional work and the social status of health professionals; how a healthcare system in which corporate interests may create more adversarial postures with health professionals will impact the way in which these groups of professionals continue to evolve, including the ultimate control and legitimacy they end up having for their work; and how changes in health professions may or may not affect societal definitions of health and illness.

There is little doubt that we are witnessing the nascent stage of profound technological innovation in healthcare delivery. At present, this innovation is occurring mainly in areas such as health information technology (e.g., electronic health records) and, slowly, in personalized healthcare (e.g., fitness apps and wearable technology used by patients). However, steady advances are being made, for example, in the use of robotics for aspects of patient care such as diagnosis and surgery, and in the use of virtual platforms to deliver care remotely. What we have seen on these fronts might be considered primitive in relation to what may be coming. Although still perhaps too early, it is well worth beginning to discuss how professional authority and work will be affected by the array of technological advances on the horizon of healthcare, driven by companies such as Google and International Business Machines (IBM).

The possibilities are endless. Even now, one could imagine a hospital, for example, with vastly fewer physicians and nurses; instead, it would be staffed by an army of robots programmed to do their tasks reliably, supplemented by strategically placed remote care devices allowing a small number of professionals to see and manage entire floors and operating rooms. Indeed, such a vision has already been seen on a small scale with technology such as centralized intensive care unit monitoring stations (Gawande, 2012). One can also imagine the use of artificial intelligence, such as IBM's Watson supercomputer, taking on the role of master diagnostician, seeking to reduce human error and improve quality in the process (Friedman, 2014). The role of all health professionals may be diminished in a future where fewer of them are required to provide care and where wider perceptions take hold regarding the fallibility of humans to make diagnosis and treatment decisions compared to the closer-to-perfection possibilities of artificial intelligence.

If this sounds like a science fiction movie, it still demands serious treatment in a number of ways, including how the professional workforce is affected. First, there likely will be a need for fewer health professionals—of all types. Second, health professionals may require new forms of training and socialization, especially in the area of continuing education, that allow them to oversee and work with the technologies placed alongside them. Third, patients, particularly younger ones who will be raised with increasingly more advanced technology in their homes and schools, may see professionals such as physicians and nurses in a diminished or more limited role, preferring instead to place their faith in the ability of various technologies to deliver their healthcare.

Those who scoff at this notion need only see the current successes of innovations such as online diagnostic (e.g., Zipnosis) and scheduling (e.g., Zocdoc) tools to imagine that new technologies with meaningful value to patients will be adopted. Even though these current technologies still place professionals at the center of their value offering, it is not hard to see how a Zipnosis, for example, might use artificial intelligence instead of a live physician to deliver diagnostic and treatment assessments to individuals and how individuals would accept these recommendations without question. As a result, the very societal legitimacy (and hence political power) of health professionals may be reduced.

Additionally, it is possible that an increasingly adversarial relationship between large, corporate-like systems and health professionals will develop, mainly as the result of tensions surrounding the cost-reduction and consumer engagement imperatives that such systems face. This results in an increasing need to view professionals as high-cost production inputs that must be managed efficiently. Although what has been discussed in this book is a future with possible accommodation, collaboration, and compromise, it is perhaps equally plausible to predict a future where tension, struggles for control, and combativeness define how health professionals coexist with their surrounding organizations.

In this latter version of the future, some of the topics of importance shift from what has been covered here and instead move into issues informed by perspectives related to dynamics such as power, politics, principal agent exchanges, and coercion. It also may shift the focus of various topics covered in this volume such as professional training, governance, leadership, and talent management, moving them in a different direction altogether. Certainly, this alternative future represents a less optimistic view than the one threaded throughout this book. However, there is enough uncertainty at present in US healthcare, in terms of how it should evolve into the future, and enough to see now in the way of increased organizational consolidation and a reduced role for individual professionals in decision-making, that such a darker scenario cannot be ruled out. At the least, it merits further analysis, especially in terms of how a professional workforce seeks to adapt, prepare, and assert itself within such a context.

Finally, and maybe most important of all, is how our very conception of health and illness are affected by an evolving health professions workforce. This topic per se was not a specific focus of the book, except in scattered doses here and there. But it looms as a critical topic for further treatment. A key question that derives from the main themes and specific content of this book is whether or not the medical model remains the dominant lens through which we as a society think about and approach the notion of healthcare. This model, which overemphasizes the curative aspects of doctoring, waiting until individuals experience symptoms for medical intervention, and the application of often expensive technological innovations to diagnose and treat existing illness, ascended to dominance through a health system ruled by physicians and the heroic nature of particular forms of their work such as surgery (Starr, 1982). In short, the medical model has defined our health system, and decision-making within it, because of the centrality of the medical profession in that system.

But the context is changing, as described here. It is fair to ask if and how certain professional dynamics might facilitate a rethinking of the medical model and, as part of that rethinking, if other paradigms for healthcare delivery can and should grow in acceptance. One alternative paradigm is that of viewing health through the lens of prevention and wellness, funneling resources and professional expertise toward service delivery aimed at keeping individuals in maximum states of good health. This minimizes the need for acute care services and higher cost specialty intervention. Related to this is a view of health and illness that emphasizes improving the social behavioral aspects of people's lives, because it is those aspects (whether or not they live in poverty or are exposed to high-stress environments in their daily lives) that have been identified as critical to keeping people from getting sick.

Some might say that a shift toward a more preventive model of health is exactly what the US healthcare system is trying to do at present, through the shifting of financial incentives toward bundled payments, innovations in primary care, and greater emphasis on things such as chronic disease management. But the counter argument is that these interventions still remain largely unable to transform in wholesale ways a system where the bulk of the profits still derive from high-cost specialty care—care that is controlled by high-prestige specialty physicians and the hospitals in which they conduct their business. Worth greater analysis is how some of the professional workforce dynamics outlined in the prior chapters might contribute to such a transformation of how we as a society think healthcare should be thought about and practiced.

Of course, there are other important issues that could be unpacked from an analysis of changes in the US health professions workforce. More of an anthology rather than an encyclopedia, this book covers only so much ground. Nevertheless, it is important ground that signifies new ways of thinking about, studying, and managing with these important workers in our healthcare system. If it stimulates further discussion, provides some with new knowledge, supports developing innovations, or provides additional grist in thinking about how to restructure the system, then it has served a meaningful purpose. Where US healthcare is presently concerned, there can be no shortage of good information or ideas, in part because it is still unclear how to make it all work in cost-effective, patient-centric, high-quality ways. Health professionals are critical to all three of these goals, which should make them a constant focus of dialogue and inquiry moving forward.

References

Abbott, A. (1988). *The system of professions*. Chicago, IL: University of Chicago Press.

Ashby, W. R. (1958). Requisite variety and its implications for the control of complex systems. *Cybernetica 1*, 83–99.

Bezrukova, K., Jehn, K. A. (2001). The effects of diversity training programs. Unpublished manuscript, Solomon Asch Center for the Study of Ethnopolitical Conflict, University of Pennsylvania, Philadelphia.

Centers for Disease Control and Prevention (CDC). (2016). *FastStats*. Retrieved from http://www.cdc.gov/nchs/fastats/physician-visits.htm.

CDC. (2014). *Health, United States, 2014*. Atlanta, GA: CDC.

Freidson, E. (1970). *Professional dominance: The social structure of medical care*. New Brunswick, NJ: Transaction Publishers.

Friedman, L. F. (April 22, 2014). IBM's Watson supercomputer may soon be the best doctor in the world. *Business Insider*. Retrieved from http://www.businessinsider.com/ibms-watson-may-soon-be-the-best-doctor-in-the-world-2014-4

Gawande, A. (August 13, 2012). Big Med: Restaurant chains have managed to combine quality control, cost control, and innovation. Can health care? *The New Yorker*. Retrieved from http://www.newyorker.com/magazine/2012/08/13/big-med

Haberstroh, C. J. (1965). Organization design and systems analysis. In J. G. March (Ed.), *Handbook of organizations* (1171–1212). Chicago, IL: Rand McNally.

Hekman, D. R., Bigley, G. A., Steensma, H. K., & Hereford, J. F. (2009). Combined effects of organizational and professional identification on the reciprocity dynamic for professional employees. *Academy of Management Journal, 52*(3), 506–526.

Hoff, T. (2005). Perceived image and utility of collective action organizations among U.S. physicians. *Research in Social Stratification and Mobility, 23*, 277–305.

Houghton Mifflin Company. (1993). *American heritage dictionary of the English language* (3rd ed). Boston, MA: Houghton Mifflin.

Institute of Medicine. (2004). *In the nation's compelling interest: Ensuring diversity in the health care workforce*. Retrieved from https://iom.nationalacademies.org/Reports/2004/In-the-Nations-Compelling-Interest-Ensuring-Diversity-in-the-Health-Care-Workforce.aspx

Jackson, S. E., Joshi, A., & Erhardt, N. L. (2003). Recent research on team and organizational diversity: SWOT analysis and implications. *Journal of Management, 29*, 801–830.

Joshi, A. (2014). By whom and when is women's expertise recognized? The interactive effects of gender education in science and engineering teams. *Administrative Science Quarterly, 59*(2), 202–239.

O'Neil, E. H., & the Pew Health Professions Commission. (1998). *Recreating health professional practice for a new century*. San Francisco, CA: Pew Health Professions Commission.

Rovner, J. (December 18, 2015). Kaiser Permanente's new medical school will focus on teamwork. *NPR*. Retrieved from http://www.npr.org/sections/health-shots/2015/12/18/460291216/kaiser-permanentes-new-medical-school-to-focus-on-teamwork

Starr, P. (1982). *The social transformation of American medicine*. New York, NY: Basic Books.

Sullivan, L. W., & the Commission on Diversity in the Healthcare Workforce. (2004). *Missing persons: Minorities in the health professions*. Retrieved from http://health-equity.pitt.edu/40/1/Sullivan_Final_Report_000.pdf

Tadelis, S. (2002). Complexity, flexibility and the make-or-buy decision. *American Economic Review, 92*(2), 433–437.

Triggle, N. (January 5, 2016). Junior doctor strikes very damaging for patients. *BBC News*. Retrieved from http://www.bbc.com/news/health-35233337

Weick, K. E., & Quinn, R. E. (1999). Organizational change and development. *Annual Review of Psychology, 50*, 361–386.

Williams, K. Y., & O'Reilly, C. (1998). Demography and diversity in organizations: A review of 40 years of research. In B. M. Staw & L. L. Cummings (Eds.), *Research in organizational behavior* (pp. 77–140). Greenwich, CT: JAI Press.

Zinn, J. S., & Brannon, S. D. (2014). Grinding strength in numbers: Bringing theoretical pluralism into the analysis of health care organizations. In S. S. F. Mick & P. D. Shay (Eds.), *Advances in health care organization theory* (2nd ed.) (53–79). San Francisco, CA: Wiley.

Index

influence on medical profession thinking,
28–29, 179
liberal insurance policies influence on, 27
medical consumption and, 27–29
support of, by outside corporate interests, 29
consumerism, 110, 131–132, 143
continuing education, 154, 165, 166, 181,
187, 193
continuous quality improvement
programs, 3, 128
control (unobtrusive), over professional
decisions
report cards, 130–131
use of peer pressure, 41, 129–131
coordinative devices of management, 123–127
cross-functional teams, 124–125
formal integrators, 123–124
liaisons, 123
matrix roles, 125–127
Core Competencies for Interprofessional Collaborative Practice (IPEC Expert Panel), 156
corporatization of healthcare delivery, 2, 24,
25–26, 47
cross-functional teams, 124

de Bruijn, H., 115
Department of Defense, 59
Department of Veterans Affairs, 59
disruptive innovations, to U.S. healthcare, 11,
29, 114–115. See also accountable care
organizations; patient-centered medical
homes; retail clinics
diversification of medical profession, implications
less predictable behavior, 35–46
reconsideration of physician power and
legitimacy, 36–39
rethinking of physician talent management
needs, 39–40
split loyalties, 36
study of assimilation vs. transformation
question, 41–42
use of different models of care, 40–41
diversity in the workplace
collaborative practices and, 74
efforts at understanding impact of, 190
gender, age, employment status, 26–27
management of, 191–192
need for embracing, 48
definitions of, 188
organizational-professional relations, 86
of physicians, in U.S. medicine,
29–35, 40–41

stratification/specialization and, 186, 189
doctor of nursing practice (DNP), 58–59
Doctor of Pharmacy (PharmD) degree, 55, 58
dyads of leadership
physicians and executives, 119–120
physicians and nurses, 120–121

ECG Management Consultants, 105
education (training) of health professionals. See
also interprofessional education
admitting process changes, 157–158
cohesive leadership role, 167
competency, defining and demonstrating,
165–166
continuing education, 154, 165, 166, 181,
187, 193
determining/disseminating best models,
165–166
Flexner Report and, 147–148, 150, 159,
161–162, 164
Frenk's report on, 150–151
gender-based graduation data, 30
Goldmark Report and, 148
key moments of change in, 147–150
length and value of, 162–163
Liaison Committee initiative for, 153–154
longitudinal integrated clerkships, 161–162
need for clarifying core competencies, 48
NP education programs, 52–53
post-1992 debt data, 27
practice-education gap, efforts at closing,
150–152
research findings on, 164–165
simulation-based education, 158–161
upskilling movement, 13, 57–59, 63, 149
electronic medical records (EMR) systems
capital requirements for, 28, 104
de-emphasis in patient-centric approach, 183
description, 10
development initiative, 3
growing necessity for, 103–104
implications of use for physicians, 9–10
role in fragmentation, 112
entrustable professional activities (EPAs), 134
evidence-based medicine movement (1970s,
1980s), 2–3

Flexner, Abraham, 147–148, 150
Flexner Report (1910), 147–148, 150, 159,
161–162, 164
formal integrators, 123–124. See also care
coordinators; hospitalists

hospital-physician relationship, 79
IHI intervention programs participation, 15
methods of integration with physicians, 127–128
new compensation methods, 86
P₄P inclusion in, 6
pharmacists' roles in, 62
professional norms, standards in, 77

IDNs. See integrated delivery networks
independent practice associations (IPAs), 112, 129
Indian Health Service, 59
Institute for Healthcare Improvement (IHI), 14–15
Institute of Medicine (IOM), 57, 110
    on absence of effective care coordination, 79
    call for interprofessional education, 153
    Future of Nursing Report, 57, 149
    on poor communication among practitioners, 155
    "To Err is Human Report," 153
integrated care practices, 26, 34, 43
    medical assistants in, 59
    NPs/PAs in, 59–60, 66–67
    payment policies, 64–65
    pharmacists in, 58, 59, 60–61
integrated delivery networks (IDNs)
    efforts at promoting, 109
    examples of, 121
    organizational compacts in, 119
    physician recruitment at, 121
integration in healthcare delivery. See also
        collaboration, interdisciplinary; leadership
        and management of healthcare workforce
    benefits of, for fragmentation, 35, 108–109, 123, 144
    challenges in achieving, 82, 109–117
    competition and, 132
    conjoint structures approach, 86–98, 104–105
    consequences of absence of, 81
    consumerism and, 110, 131–132, 143
    dyads/physicians and executives, 119–120
    dyads/physicians and nurses, 120–121
    establishing connections and, 132–133
    hospital-physician competition, role of, 132
    innovation and, 132
    leaders'/managers' roles in, 131–133
    microsystems and patient institutes, 121–122, 144
    patient centrism and, 182–183

practical considerations, 133–135
professionalism and, 131–136
societal transitions necessary for achieving, 114–116
standardization and, 131–132
theoretical considerations, 135–136
interprofessional education (IPE)
    accreditation standards, 154
    challenges of, 153–155
    defining goals for, 156–157, 173–174
    description, 152–153, 173
    IOM call for, 153
    IPEC encouragement of, 74
    Liaison Committee initiative for, 153–154
    team training and, 155–156
    WHO definition, goals for, 152–153
Interprofessional Educational Collaboration (IPEC), 74
interprofessional solidarity, 180–181
IOM. See Institute of Medicine
IPAs. See independent practice associations

Johnson & Johnson Nursing Executives Program, 129
joint collective actions, by health professionals, 180–181
Joint Commission, 14, 15, 153
Josiah Macy Jr. Foundation, 173, 174, 175
jurisdictional battles within health professions, 12–13, 35, 111–112

Kaiser Permanente, 88, 119, 121, 144, 187
Kalkman, C. J., 115

leadership and management of healthcare
        workforce. See also change, implications
        for policy, practice, management;
        collaboration, interdisciplinary;
        integration in healthcare delivery
    breaking down organizational boundaries, 122–123
    breaking down silos/overcoming divisive forces, 116–117
    challenges of collaborative models, 109–116
    changes in, 2–11
    collaboration theory and, 66
    coordinative devices, organizational tools, 123–127
    dyads/physicians and executives, 119–120
    dyads/physicians and nurses, 120–121
    efforts at breaking down boundaries, 122

pharmacists (*Cont.*)
  education upskilling, 57–59, 63, 149
  expanding scopes of practice for, 91
  expansion of pharmacy schools, 55–56
  gender-related data, 56
  hospital/hospitalist roles, 62
  importance of role of, 54
  in integrated care practices, 59–61
  need for evaluation of new roles, 65–66
  1966-2013, number and type of degrees conferred, 55
  payment policies for, 64–65
  PharmD degree, 55, 58
  regulation by state licensing boards, 56–57
  reimbursement methods, 6
  in retail clinics, 61–62
  roles in hospitals, 62
  salary arrangements, 6
  scope of practice regulations, 63–64
  self-organization by, 78
  shifting of work to, 9, 12
  utilization in various practice settings, 54–55
PharmD (Doctor of Pharmacy) degree, 55, 58
PHOs. *See* physician-hospital organizations
physical therapists, 1, 57–58, 82, 95, 149, 162, 180
physician assistants (PAs)
  comparative performance of, 60
  consumers receptivity to seeing, 51
  education upskilling, 57–59, 63
  expanding use of, 34
  gender-related data, 53–54, *54*
  healthcare spending data, 108
  historical background, 53
  in integrated care practices, 59–60
  interdependent relation with physicians, 57
  need for evaluation of new roles, 65–66
  overlapping role with NPs, physicians, 56, 65
  payment policies for, 64–65
  regulation by state licensing boards, 56
  regulatory shift towards greater independence, 57
  roles in hospitals, 62
  scope of practice of, 57
  scope of practice regulations, 63–64
  shared patient care responsibilities with younger physicians, 24–25
  shifting of work to, 9, 12
physician dominance, 43, 179–180
physician executives, 125–127
physician groups
  alignment with healthcare organizations, 92

cross-functional teams and, 124
description, 87
risk-sharing within, 86
stratification in, 23, 32
transition to "systemness" model, 104–105
physician-hospital organizations (PHOs), 83–84, 93
Physician Leadership Journal, 125
physicians. *See also* physicians, employment and integration mechanisms; physicians, younger; primary care physicians
  age, gender, specialization stratification of, 25
  attunement with retail clinics, 129
  blurring of boundaries for, 83
  burnout/well-being concerns, 48
  as central healthcare decision makers, 24
  collaboration challenges, 113–116
  consolidation alliances, 7, 26
  consumer engagement impact on, 25
  decision-making monopoly of, 107–108
  diversity in U.S. medicine, 30–34
  female vs. male conflicts, 38
  financial viability concerns, 28–29
  Flexner Report's effects on education of, 147–148, 150, 159, 161–162, 164
  hospital-physician relationship, 79
  implications of increasing diversification for, 35–42
  increasing subservience of, 28
  intraprofessional competition among, 32–33
  leadership dyad with executives, 119–120
  leadership dyad with nurses, 120–121
  licensing boards oversight of, 148
  methods of integration with hospitals, 127–128
  new breed of, 30–32
  new compensation methods, 86
  new work roles, responsibilities of, 33–34
  NPs/PAS, comparative performance, 60
  nursing's values common with, 108
  overlapping role with NPs, PAs, 56, 65
  P_4P establishment for, 5–6
  peer pressure/peer accountability by, 130
  power and legitimacy dynamics of, 36–39
  professionalism of, 107–108
  safety culture surveys of, 16
  self-organization by, 78
  shifting professional boundaries, 179–180
  talent management needs of, 39–40
  team-based care benefits for, 12–13
  transformation/internal stratification by, 25
  transition to executive roles, 125–127